Up Your Energy!

Choose Your Path To Habit Harmony

Terri Test

Up Your Energy!

Author's Note:

The content of this book is for general instruction only. Each person's physical, emotional, and spiritual condition is unique. The instruction in this book is not intended to replace or interrupt the reader's relationship with a physician or other professional. Please consult your healthcare provider for matters pertaining to your specific health and diet.

To contact the author, visit: www.balanceachieved.com

Or email:

terri@balanceachieved.com

ISBN-13: 978-0692564288

ISBN-10: 0692564284

Printed in the United States of America

This book is dedicated to my mother. You will forever be remembered for your strength, love, and tireless devotion.

Contents

Acknowledgements

To my mother, Sue; thank you for being a great listener, for tirelessly following me around on our trips to the bookstore, for being my guinea pig every time I read a new health book or article, and for sharing information with me that you learned. Most importantly, thank you for teaching me, by example, how to be a caring and compassionate individual.

To my brother, Steve, and his wife, Janeen; thank you for your daily encouragement, for sharing ideas with me, for your honest feedback, for your help with the editing, layout, and design of this book, and most importantly, for always believing in my abilities to complete this book.

Introduction

"Life is a balancing act and it isn't always necessary to make huge sacrifices to gain significant improvements."

L ife would be so much easier if your energy level kept pace with what your mind and body wanted to do. Unfortunately, there are a lot of days that you might feel as though you are making your best effort for this to happen, but somehow you fall short. You actually engage in daily habits that you think are helping to boost your energy levels, when in reality they are really zapping your energy. Sometimes you don't give your habits any thought at all and are unaware of the fact that you are actually sabotaging your energy levels.

This book is for anyone who would like to have more daily energy, may or may not know what all is causing their lower energy, feels unsure about where to begin to fix it, and wants a simple process to move forward and find a life and energy balance.

No one can keep a non-stop pace forever. At some point you have to take time to refuel your body. Sleep, water, good nutrition, and quiet time for reflection are a few of the most important ways that you can replenish the energy in your body. The way you go about refueling your body daily through the habits that you keep can either benefit your body or weaken it. Sometimes the habits you keep are well intentioned, but end up having the opposite effect than you ever expected.

Over the course of this book you will learn a simplified process for evaluating 16 daily habits that can affect your energy levels. If you are sure a particular habit is sabotaging your energy, you can jump right in and follow some or all of the simple action steps to try and modify or overcome your habit. If you aren't 100% sure that a particular habit is an issue for you, you can try one or two of the actions steps for a few weeks to see if you notice any changes in your daily energy levels.

Whether you decide to jump in with both feet or whether you do a short test drive is not important. The most important thing is that you work at being honest with yourself and take time to listen to how your body is responding to the new direction you are heading in.

This book is meant to get you thinking. We tend to put our lives on auto pilot and mindlessly go about our days—a lot of times doing the same things day in and day out without much thought. If you want more energy in your day to day life, it's time to stop running on auto pilot. It's time to start paying attention to the habits you keep and decide if they are serving you well, or if it might be time to change them up.

If you really are serious about gaining more daily energy, it is time for you to start listening to your body. It talks to you daily and gives you clues as to what isn't right. You need to learn to be a good detective by slowing down and listening to the clues. This book will help you learn how to slow down and become a good detective so that you can figure out what is in the way of you having more energy.

Each section will help you understand why it might be a good idea to evaluate each of your habits closer to see if any of them might be contributing to your energy problem. You will learn a few simple action steps to help with the process of modifying or eliminating each habit. Because everyone is individual, there are several different sets of action steps that you can take to evaluate if your habit is causing you problems. You may pick and choose which steps you want to try. What works for one may or may not work for someone else. For that reason, there is more than one set of action steps to try. Not only will you use those action steps to evaluate whether the habit is contributing to your lower energy, but you can also use the action steps to modify or eliminate your habit if you decide doing so would help improve your energy levels.

Keep in mind that once you have given one or more of your habits a serious evaluation and determined what is hindering your energy levels, you may or may not feel you have the ability to give up or modify that habit. For example, if you determine that caffeine is actually zapping your energy as opposed to boosting it up, this would mean that you may have to consider modifying how much caffeine you consume daily. For some people this may seem like an impossible habit to modify or give up. While this habit may be the best habit for you to work on, there is more than likely at least one or two other habits that you could modify or give up that may very well help your energy levels as well. You may not have to give the caffeine up if you are willing to work on the other habits instead.

Do keep in mind, though, that all habits can be modified slightly for benefits. It might not be an all or nothing process. It's about learning to live in harmony with your habits—your life and harmony balance. Everyone's place of habit harmony will be different. So just remember, you are the driving force in your own life—you decide what works for you. Sometimes just starting the process makes the next step that much easier than you ever expected.

An important thing for you to be aware of is that all of the habits described in this book have other affects on the body besides decreasing your energy levels. You may not be aware of how many benefits your body will gain by giving up or modifying any particular habit. When you choose to give up or modify one habit, you will gain at least a half a dozen or more other health benefits. This is called a synergistic effect. The Webster dictionary defines synergy as, "an effect of the interaction of the actions of two agents such that the result of the combined actions is greater than expected as a simple additive combination of the two agents acting separately." For example, a few of the added health benefits of giving up or modifying a caffeine habit are: improves sleep, may help decrease stomach acid, and may help reduce blood pressure. At the end of each habit section there is an added bonus list of other health benefits, or synergistic effects, you could receive if you modify or give up that habit.

Part One of the book is about evaluating where you are, setting small intentions to move forward, and beginning to make small but important changes in your attempt to gain more daily energy. The book describes a total of sixteen different habits that can affect your energy levels. **Part Two** describes habits that affect your Physical Health: food, nutrition, and physical body. **Part Three** describes habits that affect your Emotional Health: mind, soul, and spirituality. You may choose to skip Part One altogether and jump right into the habit sections or you may choose to go chapter by chapter evaluating what all applies to you. There is no one right way to use this book—it's all about what works for you.

Ultimately, the process of evaluating your habits and deciding whether to modify them is completely in your hands. Life is a balancing act and finding the perfect balance between your life and your habits is an ongoing process. You decide how much daily energy you need so that you can have the best life possible.

Some habits will definitely be harder to modify or break than others. If something feels really difficult, it may be because it is a really important habit for you to address. But, it also can be a sign that you aren't ready to tackle it yet. Be kind to yourself, but be honest with yourself as well. When the time is right to tackle that hard habit, you will know, you will have the resources, and you will have a better chance at being successful at it if you are truly ready to do so. Change is never easy, but sometimes necessary for you to have your best life.

Part 1

Evaluation and
Intention Setting

Chapter 1

Evaluate and Prioritize

B efore you begin your journey to find ways to have more energy, you must first take a step back and spend some time evaluating what your particular needs are. The most important resource you have is your own unique body. It talks to you on a daily basis through the good and bad symptoms that it displays. Sometimes it whispers and sometimes it silently screams at the top of its lungs. Some days it is pretty obvious what the problem or concern is. Your stomach is growling because it's hungry. Your arm is probably aching because you spent too much time on the computer. Or, your stiff neck is most likely due to spending an hour in your car commuting in busy traffic. These concerns are some of the louder cues your body gives you on a daily basis.

As you begin to evaluate some of the habits written about in this book, you will first learn to listen and pay attention to times when your body is screaming. Eventually, as you become aware of your body's cues, you will be more inclined and tuned into being able to hear the whispering as well.

Keep in mind that the screaming lets you know this is not a new problem—it is ongoing and is pretty serious at this point. Had you known how to pay closer attention to your body, you might have been able to catch the issue before it had time to get worse.

The hope is that by the time you finish working through some of the habit sections of this book, you will have a better understanding of how to listen to your body and catch your issues at the whispering stage before your issues escalate into bigger concerns.

Individual Results

Every individual will not be affected by a habit in exactly the same way. For instance, the caffeine example can be used again. Evaluating how caffeine affects you as an individual is critical. Some people can drink a few cups early in the day and not be impacted greatly. While some people have bodies that are very sensitive to caffeine and are affected if they consume even one caffeinated beverage.

You will find that some of the habits you have may require you to completely change them for you to receive the most benefit, while other habits may just require you to modify them just a little to see significant changes. What results you get from this book will depend upon several factors: how much more energy you would like to gain, how well you listen to your body, and what you are willing to actually do to see the results.

Begin an Energy Audit

For you to know what is really having an impact on your energy levels, you have to spend a little time evaluating where you are. So many people rush through life doing the same things daily, never noticing what actions they may be taking that might be contributing to their decreased energy levels. This doesn't have to be a complicated process, but it does need to be somewhat detailed.

For you to understand where your energy issues are, you must first start paying close attention to what you are doing every day that might be affecting your levels. There are a few different ways you can keep track of this information. You can purchase a small notebook to write notes in daily, use a word document program on your computer, or use a note taking program on your phone. The most important thing is that you use some kind of system to keep track daily of this information.

The purpose of the energy audit is to keep track of your food, activity, and thinking done daily so that you can decide what activities your lower energy issues may be associated with. You can write down information throughout the day or you can sit down in the evening and write out everything you remember about the day. Keep the process simple, but try to notice as many details about your days and how you are feeling with respect to your energy levels.

Depending upon how your schedule changes weekly will determine how long you will need to do this process. If your schedule changes every week, you may need to do this for several weeks. But if your schedule is exactly the same each week, you may only need to do your energy audit for a week or two.

You are looking for patterns during your day when your energy is higher at one point and lower at another. When you have a different experience one day or even a part of a day, you want to know what was different about that day that contributed to your worse or better energy levels. Keep in mind there is no right or wrong way to do this process. The more in tune you become with your body, the more benefit you will get from this process.

Here are some questions to ask yourself.

(Note: To find a printable copy of all of the Energy Audit questions go to www.balanceachieved.com)

In the Morning:

Did you start off the day with energy — feeling rested?

Did you indulge in a pick-me-up? (Example: coffee.) What and When?

Did you eat breakfast? If so, what did you eat and when did you eat it?

Did you spend any quiet time meditating?

Mid Morning:

Did you eat a snack? If so, what was the snack?

Did you feel the need for a pick-me-up? What did you have and when?

Were you more tired at this point than earlier?

At Lunch:

Did you eat lunch? If so, what did you eat?

Did you feel the need for another pick-me-up? If you had something, what and when did you have it?

Where is your energy level at this point?

How much time did you spend at lunch?

Mid Afternoon:

Did you eat an afternoon snack? If so, what did you eat?

Did you feel the need for a pick-me-up? What did you have and when?

Did you feel like you wanted a nap?

How is your energy level at this point compared to earlier in the day?

What activities were you doing at this time?

At Dinner:

Did you eat dinner? If so, what did you eat and when did you eat it?

How is your energy at this point?

After Dinner:

Did you have a snack or dessert after dinner? If so, what did you eat and when did you eat it?

What activities did you do after dinner? List all with times.

Did you spend any quiet time for reflecting or doing something you enjoy? If so, what did you do and for how long?

How was your energy level at this point?

Recap of Yesterday:

Did you work yesterday? If so, what time frame?

Did you exercise at any time during the day? If so, what did you do and for how long?

Did you consume any caffeinated drinks after 3:00 pm? If so, what, and how much did you have?

What time did you go to bed and how many hours of sleep did you get?

Did you feel rested when you woke in the morning or did you wake up a lot during the night?

Did you do anything for your own self-care? (Examples: read, go to a social event, watch sports, or get a massage.)

What people did you have interactions with during the day? List them all.

For each interaction, rate the encounter from 1 to 10 with 10 being a very happy and positive interaction.

Evaluating your Findings

Once you have collected all the energy audit material, you should begin to see patterns of when you have energy, when you don't, and what things might be contributing in a positive way and what in a negative way. For instance, if you had more energy on two days of the week, but not the rest of the work week, look for why. Maybe you got an extra hour of sleep on each of the two better days and you noticed you didn't need as many pick-me-ups those days either. Maybe on two days you had really low energy in the afternoon and upon further investigation, you noticed that you didn't eat any breakfast on either of those days. Maybe you noticed that you didn't sleep well on two different nights. On further evaluation, you realize you ate a candy bar each of the two nights before bedtime and you had a disagreement with your significant other both nights as well.

The most important take away here is that you have to look for patterns of behavior that lead to negative results. It's so easy to just push through your day to get it over with never stopping to take notice of what habits you are continually taking part in. If you really want to get to the root cause of your energy issue, you have to learn to take notice of everything you do during your waking hours.

Prioritize

The next part of the process is entirely up to you. Once you know what seems to be your issues — not enough sleep, indulging in too many pick-me-ups, not having enough good interactions, or whatever the case may be, you can take this information and begin looking into the habit sections to see what habits might be issues for you to work on. The habits in this book are divided into two main categories of your life: **Physical Health** (food, nutrition, and physical body) and **Emotional Health** (mind, soul, and spirituality).

You may decide that there is one main area you would like to evaluate further or you may decide that there are several areas you would like to look into.

If you do decide that you would like to look into more than one area, prioritize them. List them on a piece of paper and next to each, rank the order of importance to you. Once you have chosen which habit you would

like to work on first, you can move on to **Chapter 2.**
Save this list and know that at anytime you can come
back and begin working on the next listed habit.

Chapter 2

Set Small Intentions

Once you know what habit you would like to take a closer look at first, spend some time looking over the individual section. Read about the possible action steps that you can take to further evaluate whether that habit is a significant energy zapper for you. Spend a week or two actually trying out some of the action steps to see if you see any difference in your energy levels over that time period. If you do notice a difference, that particular habit may be one you want to actually modify or eliminate all together.

Remember to start out working on only one habit at a time. It's important to not over commit. You don't want to set yourself up for failure. Be really patient with yourself and realize that you didn't gain the habit over night so you won't modify or eliminate it without putting in some time and dedication. Remember that it takes at least 21 days to create a new habit. If you are trying to eliminate an old habit, you are basically trying to create a new life habit.

Once you have chosen a habit to modify or eliminate, decide what your approach will be. Will you follow one or more of the action steps in the book or will you choose another method of your own? Do you want to work on this every day of the week, or will you initially work on it a few days out of the week and then increase your time? Set a small intention, write it out, post the intention somewhere to remind yourself of the commitment, or tell a friend or family member to hold you accountable for it.

For example, if you wanted to change your habit of trading sleep for awake time you might decide that your intention is to work on getting more sleep on Sundays and Wednesdays because those are the nights you tend to stay up extra hours. After evaluating all the possible action steps, you decide that you will make sure you exercise either early in the morning or right after work so it won't affect your sleep. You also decide that you will record your favorite television shows on those nights so you can get in the bed at 10:00 p.m. You also set an intention to try this new behavior for one month and then re-evaluate how you feel after that.

Adding New Intentions

If you decide you see some results, but not enough, you may need to commit to more changes. Using the sleep example above, you may decide that you need to work on getting more sleep on more days per week, or you may decide that you are more concerned about what is affecting the quality of your sleep, not just the quantity. At this point, you can add in a few more actions steps or make an appointment and have a discussion with your healthcare provider.

Switching to a New Habit

If you get some results from modifying or eliminating one habit, but you still feel like your energy level isn't where you would like it to be, you can consider evaluating another habit. Go back to the list you created in **Chapter 1** and begin the evaluation process for habit #2 on your list. Read over that habit section in the book and do a week or two evaluation of that habit to see if you see a difference in your daily energy. If you do see a difference, start the process over and set a new intention for the second habit that you have decided to work on. Continue this process for every new habit you choose to work on.

Part 2

Physical Health Habits

Depending on Caffeine as Your Pick-Me-Up

It may be difficult to hear this, but to be fair and balanced when evaluating habits that contribute to decreased energy, you have no choice but to look at your consumption of caffeine. Whether your caffeine comes from coffee, tea, soda, or an energy drink, it doesn't matter. What matters is how much caffeine you actually consume and what else is in your drink— primarily the concern would be if it is loaded with a lot of sugar or artificial sweeteners.

Let's talk about coffee first. If you have this habit, you certainly have lots of company. The continued success of the coffee industry is about as much proof of that as you need. While some experts and studies argue that there are health benefits to coffee, there are others arguing that it is a huge energy zapper. If that isn't confusing enough, there is yet a third body of experts that argue that coffee is okay if consumed in moderation. It isn't your cup of Joe that is creating all of your energy issues. It's the total amount of caffeine you are consuming daily and how much and what additives are in each daily cup. There is definitely a huge difference between a cup of black coffee and a double shot vanilla latte.

If soda, energy drinks, or sports drinks are your drinks of choice, the same applies to these regarding the caffeine. If you look at your labels, you may find that these carry as much or more caffeine as any coffee drink you get. What could be different here, depending upon your preferences of coffee drinks, is the amount of sugar added. A lot of these types of drinks are loaded with added sugar. Whether we are talking about natural cane sugar or artificial sweeteners, the jury isn't out at all on this matter. Most all experts agree—sugar, in any form, should only be consumed in a very moderate amount. To understand more how sugar affects your energy, read the two sections in this book titled: "Giving in to Your Sugar Cravings" and "Overlooking your Blood Sugar Swings."

If tea is your caffeinated drink of choice, you definitely won't have as many critics. Tea does have a lot of health benefits and most of the time has less caffeine than other choices. If you are a tea drinker, and you think you may have a caffeine issue, take a look at how much caffeine is actually in each cup. Some types of tea do have more caffeine than others. Also, look at how much added sugar is in it—whether you are adding your own sugar in or whether you purchase a drink that has it added already.

In order for you to figure out whether caffeine is affecting you or not, you have to take a step back and evaluate where your energy level currently is and where you would like it to be. If caffeine is having an impact on your energy, it might not be easy to admit to yourself. So many people use caffeine as a late morning or early afternoon pick-me-up on a daily basis. Others like the ritual of holding that cup of coffee or can of soda in their hand first thing in the morning and feel like they need that boost to get their day off to the right start. Why you choose to indulge in caffeine doesn't matter. What matters is that you be honest with yourself on how caffeine is affecting your particular body. Coffee, tea, soda, and energy drinks are temporary solutions to keeping you going.

Some peoples' bodies are much more sensitive than others on how caffeine affects them. It's important to figure out if your body is more sensitive to it than you realized. Bottom line, it never hurts to remember that everything in moderation is always better than consistently over indulging in anything. And, while coffee, tea, soda, and energy or sports drinks do count toward your daily fluid intake, the more you drink of them, the less water you are drinking. Ultimately, it is important to remember that water always trumps any other drink choice you can make.

Evaluate Your Intake

If you want to figure out whether caffeine is affecting your energy, spend a week or two taking notes on your caffeine intake and how you feel throughout each day. It is important for you to look at how many milligrams of caffeine are actually in each drink you consume. Because some people are more sensitive to caffeine than others, this could be very important information. Write down how much added sugar you put into the drink you fix yourself, or look at the label of what you purchase and figure out what the added sugar amounts to. Track how you are feeling before you consume the drink and evaluate how you are feeling one or two hours after you finish the drink. Did you start out in a neutral place, then gain some energy, and then feel like you crashed a little? Did you feel the need to grab a pick-me-up midmorning or mid afternoon? How was your mood throughout the day? What was the exact time you consumed your last caffeinated beverage?

Because it is considered a chemical stimulant, understanding how long it takes for caffeine to be eliminated from your system is important to know. The elimination process for drugs and chemicals is measured by something called a half-life. The half-life is the time required for the amount of the drug or chemical to fall to half of its initial value. The half-life of caffeine can be anywhere from six to eight hours depending upon who consumes it. For example, the half-life could actually be less time for a smoker and more time for a pregnant woman. If you consume any caffeine after 3:00 pm in the afternoon, there is a good chance it won't be completely eliminated from your system by bedtime and could ultimately alter the quality of sleep of a more sensitive person. For this reason it is important to pay attention to how your sleep is each night with respect to the caffeine you drink.

There are a few more sources of caffeine that a lot of people forget about, but need to be noted in your caffeine totals. Some medications as well as weight control products have added caffeine as does your favorite source of chocolate—whether that be in the form of candy or some other delicious chocolaty treat. Make sure you check out the packaging and include this in your daily caffeine intake totals. Once you take note of how much you are truly consuming daily, including how much added sugar you are getting, then it will be easier for you to decide if this is an energy zapper for you versus an energy provider for you. You may just need to modify your habit slightly to see significant results.

(Note: Decaf coffee does have caffeine in it so make sure you add this to your totals.)

Consider a Decrease

If you think you are consuming too many milligrams of caffeine per day, consider decreasing the amount. You can do this several ways. If you usually drink three cups of coffee per day, drop down to two cups a day and drink a caffeine-free or lower caffeine beverage in place of one of your cups of coffee. You can also look at the type of coffee you drink most often and the way the coffee is prepared. Some types of coffee are naturally higher in caffeine than others. The finer you grind the coffee, the more caffeine is released, and the more grounds you put in your coffee maker, the more caffeine you will get per cup. You can also do a mix of your favorite coffee blend and a lower caffeinated blend.

For soda or energy drink lovers, pay attention to your labels. Try drinking one less can per day. If you miss the one you take away, add in a can of something with less sugar and less caffeine. If you are up for it, switch out all of your daily cans with a lower sugar and less caffeinated beverage. Even though it may be tempting, never chose a product with less caffeine, but more sugar — added sugar is never a better option.

For tea drinkers, look at the caffeine content of what you drink. Also pay attention to the extra sugar you add or the manufacturer adds. Change to another kind of tea that has less caffeine. Consider brewing the tea a little less time so there is less caffeine in it. If you brew your own tea bags for iced tea, mix one regular bag of black tea with one bag of herb tea. Experiment with different flavors until you find a combination you enjoy.

Try One Day on and One Day Off

Take a look at how many days per week you drink a caffeinated beverage. If you drink some form of caffeine every day, consider taking a day off. If the half-life of one caffeinated beverage is, on average, six to eight hours, think about what happens when you add one or two more beverages into the mix. Your body is processing even more caffeine over a 24 hour period of time and by the time you start your next day, you might be adding more caffeine on top of yesterday's caffeine depending upon how late in the day you consumed it and how sensitive your body is to caffeine. Try one day on and one day off or two days on and one day off. For the off days, try adding in a caffeine free substitute.

Make a Caffeine Swap

There are a lot of low or no caffeine alternatives on the market. Swaps for no caffeine beverages could include: roasted grain coffees, herbal coffees, herbal tea, caffeine free soda, flavored water, sparkling water with fresh fruit, flavored seltzer water, or even fresh juice.

Swaps for less caffeine beverages could include: kombucha, decaffeinated coffee, instant coffee, green tea, yerba mate, black tea, decaffeinated tea, Darjeeling white tea, or hot chocolate. You could visit your local health food store and see what options are available, ask your favorite coffee shop barista for options, or search the internet for new items to try.

Synergistic effects of not depending on caffeine as your pick-me-up:

- Improves sleep
- May help decrease stomach acidity
- May help reduce blood pressure
- May help decrease inflammation
- Helps maintain more stable blood sugar levels
- Decreases risk for osteoporosis
- Decreases risk for dehydration

Habit **TWO**_____

Being Addicted to Carbohydrates

Carbohydrates are an extremely important part of your daily diet. They provide the body with glucose—your body's main source of dietary energy. While no one will argue the fact that they are an important part of your daily diet, the main take away here is that all carbohydrates are not created equal. When it comes to giving you sustained energy throughout your day, some are better than others.

There are two main kinds of carbohydrates classified by how the body breaks them down. The first category of carbohydrates is called simple carbohydrates or simple sugars. They are called simple because they are quickly broken down by the body to release energy. An example of a simple carbohydrate food is a donut. The second category of carbohydrates is referred to as complex carbohydrates. They are made up of hundreds of simple carbohydrates and are broken down more slowly and provide a slower, steadier release of energy for the body. An example of a complex carbohydrate is a serving of beans.

The healthiest carbohydrate choices are complex carbohydrates—fresh fruits and vegetables, whole grains, and beans—these provide the body with vitamins, minerals, fiber, and other phytonutrients and are broken down more slowly providing the body with a slower and steadier release of energy.

The unhealthier choices of carbohydrates are simple carbohydrates—white bread, pastries, white rice, and other processed or refined foods.

If you are having a lot of energy issues, you may need to look at the quality of the carbohydrates you are consuming daily. It is very important to balance your daily diet so that you eat evenly over the course of the day—breakfast, lunch, and dinner as well as one snack midmorning and one snack mid to late afternoon. It is also important to add in protein and a serving of good fat with each main meal as well. The more you balance your meals throughout the day, the less often your blood sugar will spike and then crash later causing huge fluctuations in your energy levels.

Keep in mind that every individual has different needs when it comes to how many carbohydrates are needed daily. Generally speaking, men need more than women and the more active you are, especially those who are athletes, the more carbohydrates you will need to consume daily. If you have any major health issues or chronic diseases, you will need to discuss what your particular daily carbohydrate needs are with your healthcare provider.

NOTE: Make sure you also read the section in this book on "Overlooking Your Blood Sugar Swings." This section will give you more suggestions on how to work on this habit. The most important take away is that you need to eat balanced meals — not all carbohydrates, not all protein — but a good mix of both with some good fat added in to each meal as well. Possible protein sources are: eggs, fish, lean meat, dairy foods, or vegetarian alternatives such as soy protein powder, whey protein powder, soybeans, tofu, or tempeh. Some healthy fat sources are: avocado, seeds, nuts, olive oil, or salmon.

Journal What You Eat Daily

You may not be aware of how many carbohydrates you consume or whether they are considered simple or complex. Spend a few days writing down every food you eat. Also write down how you were feeling at the time you ate each food and how you felt an hour or more later. Ask yourself why you ate what you ate. Were you hungry? Were you stressed? Were you bored? If you ate for any other reason than hunger, make sure you check out the section in this book on "Overlooking the Fact That You Overeat."

Find a food chart and look up the number of carbohydrates that are in each of the food items that you consumed. Decide if each food is considered a simple or a complex carbohydrate. Also, take note of how many times a day you eat and whether or not some foods actually sustain your energy and hunger longer than others. Keep any food items in your meal plans if they do help with your hunger and sustain your energy levels.

Once you know what you eat, when you eat it, and how you feel after you eat it, you can decide where you need to make changes in your diet.

Learn to Read Labels

One of the best ways to improve your overall health and energy levels is to learn to read food labels. Unless you are only eating fresh fruits and vegetables, everything you consume will have a food label on it. Some products will have very few extra ingredients, but most packaged products will have a bunch of extra additives. Initially, focus on learning the main information on the label—servings per container, calories, fat, sodium, carbohydrates, fiber, sugar, and protein. For the purposes of this book, not all of these nutritional items will be referred to, but the more you begin to pay attention to them all, the more you will learn which packaged items you eat are better choices overall.

If you work at trying to balance your meals throughout the day, by eating fiber rich carbohydrates and quality protein with every meal, you may find that you have more sustained energy because your blood sugar levels will not spike and dip as much. If you want to know what the nutritional information on your broccoli is, you can look for charts online or purchase a small pocket guide. Remember that carbohydrates in the form of fresh fruits and vegetables are the better way to eat, but the amount of carbohydrates and fiber in each different fruit and vegetable can vary quite a bit as well.

As a basic guide, try to eat a balance of 2 to 1 for your carbohydrates to protein ratio per meal. An example of that would be if you eat a piece of chicken that has 24 grams of protein, try to keep your carbohydrate level at or preferably below 48 grams—that is one part protein to 2 parts carbohydrates. (Remember—if you have any major health issues, or chronic diseases, speak with your healthcare provider on what a good ratio of protein and carbohydrates are for you.)

Something else to be aware of is what the Glycemic Index or (GI) rating is for the carbohydrate. Lower ranked GI foods can have less of an impact on blood sugar levels than high ranked GI foods. You can find books on the glycemic index and charts with the ratings of most of the common foods consumed. Focusing on eating primarily low GI rating foods may help with your energy levels as well. Do a vegetable swap and journal if you see any differences in how you feel eating one item over another.

Another thing to pay close attention to is the sugar content in your foods. So many packaged or canned foods have sugar added for more flavor. One teaspoon of sugar is equal to four grams of sugar. So if you eat a candy bar that has 24 grams of sugar, you are consuming 6 teaspoons of sugar in that one candy bar. (The math on that—24 grams divided by 4 grams per teaspoon equals 6 teaspoons of sugar.) Some nutritionists will tell you that you probably shouldn't have much more sugar than that, if any, in an entire day.

You will tend to notice that your simple carbohydrates, like the candy bar, will break down quicker in the body causing the spikes in blood sugar levels—leading to energy dips. Complex carbohydrates (like whole grain breads, brown rice, and quinoa) paired with good fats, protein, and fiber will break down slower and give the body more of a chance to deal with the sugars more gradually. If you choose natural foods over processed foods you will notice a difference in how your body deals with them as well.

Pack Your Snacks

It is so easy to grab a bag of chips or a candy bar out of that vending machine when you feel that mid morning or mid afternoon slump. Planning ahead and purchasing more quality items for those times will keep you from having those energy crashes. One suggestion is to buy a large container of mixed nuts and fill small snack bags with a handful. This is easy to keep in the car, your purse, or in your desk drawer — and you don't have to worry about them spoiling right away. You can also cut up vegetables and bring a little container of hummus or pack a cup of cottage cheese and have a piece of fruit with it. There are lots of quality snacks that will keep your blood sugar levels more balanced so that you won't have energy dips throughout your day. Make it your intention to come up with several snack ideas that are easy for you to prepare and take with you every day.

Try Eating the Bulk of Your Carbohydrates Early in the Day

Figuring out why you don't have the energy you need throughout each day is all about listening to your body and playing detective. Sometimes you will uncover clues that are obvious and sometimes you will have to dig a little deeper. If at some point you feel like you are balancing your food at every meal, but you still are feeling like your energy level isn't where you would like it to be, try something different with your carbohydrates. Try consuming the majority of them in only the first part of your day. Set an intention that after 3:00 pm every day you will only consume carbohydrates in the form of fresh vegetables. Plan dinners that consist of only protein and fresh vegetables—no pasta, rice, potatoes, bread, or dessert. Plan on eating fruit before 3:00 pm. Try this process for at least a week and journal what you eat, how you feel, and how much energy you have.

Watch Your Drinks

Water should be the main drink everyone has daily, but the reality is, some days it isn't. The energy drink you grab mid morning or mid afternoon, or the coffee drink you grab on the way to work can be loaded with carbohydrates and sugar.

When you are doing your journaling for the foods you eat daily, make sure you also write down the drinks you consume throughout the day. Read the nutritional information on the next can you grab or the next coffee drink you order. How many carbohydrates does it have versus protein that it offers? Is it fairly balanced or are there a lot more carbohydrates than protein? Notice how you feel an hour or so after you drink it. Do you seem to get a huge burst of energy and then dip an hour or two later? Remember, the goal is for sustained energy throughout your day. It might be time to rethink that drink.

Do Food Swaps

Some people are more sensitive to carbohydrates than others. Because you need good quality carbohydrates to fuel your body, you don't want to stop eating them. What you may want to focus on instead is finding ways to make healthier choices — choosing items that don't spike your blood sugar levels as much.

Eating a donut is definitely going to spike your blood sugar levels. But trading the donut for a high protein snack bar can give your taste buds something chewy, a little bit of sweet, a good amount of protein, and a much better chance you won't have blood sugar levels that crash an hour or so later.

Make a list of the carbohydrates you eat regularly that aren't the best choices. Begin to search for healthier swaps that will help keep your blood sugar levels more stable. There are lots of recipes on the internet and great ideas for swaps as well. There are also a lot of cookbooks available with better quality carbohydrate recipes for main dishes as well as desserts and snacks.

Do remember that it is still important to read labels. Don't assume that a high fiber fruit muffin will be a good swap for a donut unless you have read the ingredient list and know for sure what the nutritional chart says.

Keep in mind that this process of evaluating your carbohydrates isn't necessarily about eating a low carbohydrate diet. It is about choosing better quality carbohydrates on a more consistent basis. It is okay to splurge, but if you do it every day, you won't be able to keep good energy levels consistently.

Cravings Don't Seem to be Budging

If you try several of these ideas and also some of the ideas in the "Overlooking Your Blood Sugar Swings" section, and you still see no huge changes, it may be time to visit your healthcare provider. Sometimes carbohydrate cravings are a sign of nutritional deficiencies in your body. Your body may be deficient in B vitamins, magnesium, chromium, or other vitamins or minerals. You could also be battling a bout of depression. Your healthcare provider can do some lab work and help you figure out if there are any other health issues you should be concerned with that are making you crave carbohydrates and keeping your energy levels down.

Synergistic effects of not being a carbohydrate addict:

- Decreases brain fog
- Helps maintain more stable blood sugar levels
- Improves fat burning process
- Improves sleep
- Aids in fewer cravings
- Helps maintain a strong immune system
- Decreases risk for chronic diseases

Overlooking Your Blood Sugar Swings

Whether you are a diabetic or not, keeping your blood sugar balanced throughout the day is important to maintain a good, consistent energy level. To do this you need to eat the right balance of foods throughout the day so that you are not having spikes and dips in your blood sugar levels. Skipping meals or not eating the right balance of protein and carbohydrates will cause your blood sugar levels to fluctuate over the course of the day. Not only will you see a decrease in energy, but you might also see signs like: headaches, nausea, blurred vision, shakiness, and trouble concentrating – depending upon whether your blood sugar is spiking or dipping.

The best way to keep your blood sugar balanced is to eat breakfast, lunch, dinner and two quality snacks in between. As a general rule, try to eat within 1 hour of rising in the morning and space your meals and snacks out so that you are consuming food about every 2 ½ to 3 hours.

Another important reason to have that afternoon snack is that around 4:00 pm your blood sugar, serotonin, and mood have a tendency to plummet. If you don't have that afternoon snack, you might have a tendency to overeat at dinner which can affect your sleep later that night and could potentially lead to you gaining more weight.

Keep a Food Journal

Spend a week writing down everything that you eat throughout each day. Log every snack, treat, drink, glass of water, and even write down that glass of wine you consume while cooking dinner. At the end of each day, figure out how much protein, fiber, and carbohydrates you are consuming. Write down how you felt during the day after you consumed that meal, snack, or drink. Did you feel energized at first? Did you feel like your energy plummeted a few hours later? Where you able to concentrate more during certain parts of the day? What food did you consume around the times you did better? What food did you consume when you felt worse? This food log will help you to figure out where you might be getting it right and where you might need to change it up so that you can have more consistent energy throughout your entire day—not just part of the day.

Balance Your Protein and Carbohydrates

A quick rule of thumb is to never have a meal or snack that doesn't have a good balance between the carbohydrates and the protein —try for a ratio of 2 to 1.

Read food labels or look at a food chart to learn how many carbohydrates the vegetables, fruit, and grains you eat have in them. Also, check out how much protein is in the meat, soy, or dairy products that you are consuming. For example: if you are going to eat a small piece of chicken that has 24 grams of protein, you want the carbohydrates you consume to be no more than twice your total protein or 48 grams for the carbohydrates. Keep in mind that 48 grams of carbohydrates would be considered on the high side for the balance of this particular meal and choosing to consume foods with a lot less carbohydrates would be better with regards to balancing your blood sugars.

Something else that helps to offset your carbohydrates is fiber. The more fiber in your meal, the more it helps, along with the protein, to balance your meal.

The easiest way to remember this formula is to take the protein you are eating, double it, and know that your carbohydrates should always be less than that doubled number.

If you enjoy eating a bowl of oatmeal for breakfast, you will have to add other items to the meal so that there will be a good balance of carbohydrates and protein. The oatmeal container states that there are 26 grams of carbohydrates and 5 grams of protein per ½ cup. If you double the protein total, that would be 10 grams. That is still very short of having a good carbohydrate and protein balance. For this meal to be more balanced, you need to add a minimum of 8 more grams of protein for there to be a 2 to 1 ratio—5 plus 8 grams of protein would be 13 grams of protein which when doubled is 26. You will have to mix several higher protein items into the oatmeal or eat a higher protein item alongside the oatmeal so that it is a more balanced meal.

Possible protein sources are: eggs, fish, lean meat, dairy food, or a vegetarian alternative such as soy protein powder, whey protein powder, soybeans, tofu, or tempeh. Beans are another source of protein and fiber, but they do have more carbohydrates. For this reason, beans might not be your first choice depending upon what else you eat alongside them.

A general rule is to have a piece of lean meat the size of the palm of your hand or no bigger than a deck of cards. If you are a vegetarian, you will have to pay close attention to your meals and make sure you also add the appropriate amount of plant based protein. The amount of protein grams you need daily depends upon your body size and activity level. If you are unsure of how much protein you should be eating, have a discussion with your healthcare provider. The bulk of protein you consume will be with each of your three main meals, but your snacks should have a smaller balance of protein and carbohydrates as well.

Focus On Eating Low-GI Foods

Understand that all carbohydrates are not created equal. In 1981, Dr. David Jenkins, along with a team of researchers at the University of Toronto, created a system to manage blood sugar levels called the glycemic index (GI).

This system ranks foods that contain carbohydrates into categories of low, medium, or high and works off of a scale of 1 to 100 with 1 being the lowest GI ranking and 100 being the highest GI ranking. Low GI foods (with a ranking of 0-55) produce little to no fluctuations in your blood sugar and insulin levels. Foods with a high GI ranking which include items such as—white rice, potatoes, most breads and pastries, watermelon, most cereals, beets, and cake—rapidly raise blood sugar levels.

Food containing good quality carbohydrates that are rich in fiber and nutrients help your body feel full, keep you alert, and help sustain your energy level throughout the day. Some carbohydrates break down slow and some a little faster. The slower they break down after you eat them, the longer your blood sugar levels will stay stable and not fluctuate. Consider eating foods that have a low glycemic index rating to help with this concern. There are many books and internet resources available for you to research to find out which foods tend to be better choices with regards to their GI level.

(Also, refer to the section in the book titled, "Being Addicted to Carbohydrates" to better understand the two different forms of carbohydrates.)

Don't Skip Breakfast

If you want to get your day off to the right start, make sure you have a high protein breakfast within one hour of rising. If you skip breakfast, you are setting your body up for a roller coaster ride with respect to your blood sugar levels throughout the day. If you change nothing else about your eating habits, make sure you eat a high protein breakfast every day. If you don't feel like eating anything, try drinking a smoothie with protein powder. A smoothie is an easy way to get a protein rich meal. It can also be a good option for lunch as well. If you opt for the smoothie, make sure you watch how much fruit or added sugar goes into it or you could still have blood sugar issues. Watch the GI levels of your fruits as well.

Watch your Pick-Me-Ups

Start reading the labels on those drinks or snacks you grab to help with your energy slumps. Snacks out of a vending machine, the coffee treat from your local coffee shop, and those energy drinks you purchase from the convenience store are usually loaded with a ton of sugar. Food labels list sugar in grams. One teaspoon of sugar is equivalent to 4 grams of sugar. The American Heart Association recommends the upper limit of your daily sugar intake be 6 teaspoons per day for women (or 24 grams) and 9 teaspoons per day for men (or 36 grams). Some health professionals will argue that even that is too much sugar.

If your drink or snack says it has 12 grams of sugar, you are consuming 3 teaspoons of sugar in one item. That is half of the days recommended allowance per the American Heart Association Guidelines if you are a woman. The more sugar you are consuming with each meal or snack with no regards to balancing the protein and carbohydrates in it, the more your blood sugar levels will spike and then dip a few hours later. Instead of grabbing those sugary treats, snack on a handful of nuts, some hummus and vegetables, a good quality protein bar, or some kind of nut butter and apple slices. Do an internet search for healthy high protein snack ideas and start packing snacks to take with you every day so your blood sugar levels will stay more balanced.

Synergistic effects of keeping your blood sugar balanced:

- Decreases brain fog
- Aids in fewer cravings/hunger
- Improves ability to exercise
- Improves sleep
- Helps maintain more stable moods
- Aids in fewer PMS symptoms
- Aids in fewer hot flashes
- Reduces risk for diabetes
- Reduces risk for heart disease
- Improves fat burning process
- Reduces risk for kidney disease

Giving In To Sugar Cravings

Having an occasional sweet treat is not a problem. Consuming foods daily that contain a lot of sugar, on the other hand, is a huge energy zapper. If you crave sugar and find yourself reaching for it several times a day, you are going to have to take a step back and seriously evaluate why you need to do this.

The sneaky part about sugar is that initially you feel energized because it spikes your blood sugar levels. But, if you will pay close attention to your body the next time you consume it, you will also notice how non-energized and tired you feel a short time later depending upon how much sugar you had and what your other meals that day were like. This occurs because your blood sugar levels then take a huge dip.

Your goal daily is to have study blood sugar levels throughout your day, not ones that skyrocket and plummet several times a day like a crazy roller coaster ride.

This can be a challenging habit to overcome, but it can be done if you set your mind to it, be patient with yourself, and work on simple, daily changes.

Read Food Labels

If you really want to cut out some of the sugar in your diet, start reading food labels. So many companies sneak sugar into their products for enhanced flavor.

Packaged products such as spaghetti sauce, soup, bread, crackers, and even lunch meat have added sugar in them for improved flavor. Dairy products have natural sugar in them, but some products such as fruit flavored yogurts add a ton more sugar for flavor as well. Take a look at the label on the bottle of your favorite juice. Make sure that it is 100% juice and that there is no added sugar.

Another way food manufacturers sneak sugar in is by calling sugar by a different name—fructose, dextrose, malt syrup, sucrose, high-fructose corn syrup, and maltose are just a few names that are used.

Start out by learning to read the labels of the food packages you currently have at home. Look at the ingredient list for that drink you purchase every day. Look at the label on the snack bar you buy from the vending machine. Take note of all the regular items you put into your grocery cart each week. You have to become familiar with what you do daily so you can decide if you need to make any changes.

Create a Visual Picture

There are four grams of sugar in one teaspoon. If your energy drink says that it has 18 grams of sugar, then that is equal to 18 divided by 4 grams or 4 ½ teaspoons of sugar. Spend an entire day journaling every food item you eat for the day. Next to each item that you journal, write down how much sugar is in it. (Convert all grams of sugar to teaspoons.)

Make sure you include the sugar that you add to your morning cup of coffee or bowl of oatmeal as well. Remember, you are focusing on only items that sugar doesn't come in naturally — where a manufacturer or food preparer added sugar to an item so that it would be more flavorful. Take notice of added sugar in packaged food items like: spaghetti sauce, flavored yogurt, breakfast cereal, granola bars, bread, lunch meat, chips, crackers, and canned soup.

Once you have written down all the food you ate for the day and listed the sugar totals, add them all up. Take a tall, clear drinking glass and fill it up with the exact amount of teaspoons of sugar that you consumed that day. Seeing how full your glass is with sugar will help you to be aware of how much sugar you truly consume on a daily basis.

The American Heart Association recommends that added sugar be limited in daily diets to: up to 6 teaspoons of sugar per day for women and up to 9 teaspoons of sugar per day for men. If a woman were to have consumed the energy drink mentioned above, she would have consumed over half of her suggested daily total of sugar by drinking just that one energy drink.

Start with Your Drinks

One of the easiest ways to cut out sugar is to look at what you are drinking daily. If you are drinking anything other than water, chances are you could be consuming more sugar than you realize. (This should be more obvious to you now after the above energy drink example.)

Pre-packaged drinks like soda, sports drinks, energy drinks, and even juices have a lot of added sugar. Read your labels and know how much you are consuming daily. If you only drink these items occasionally, it isn't as big of a concern for your energy levels. But, if you consume them on a daily basis, you can bet your energy levels are taking a big hit.

Other drinks that people commonly have daily are usually some kind of coffee beverage. This might actually be a better choice because you have a lot more control over how much sugar goes into it. You can control how much sugar the barista puts in your drink or how many teaspoons of sugar that you add to it.

Make an effort to learn how much sugar is added into the drink you buy. Most restaurants have websites with nutritional information and some restaurants actually have a printed version on hand for consumers to look at as well.

Once you know what you consume daily, you can decide on ways to decrease your sugary drinks. You might: choose different products with less sugar, be aware of how much sugar goes into your coffee beverage, or stop drinking the products all together and choose water or iced tea instead.

The goal here is to make a gradual switch so that your taste buds will slowly get used to less sugar. Before you know it, the old favorites you used to drink will taste too sweet.

Substitute Healthier Sweeteners

There is a lot of controversy on which products are safer and healthier choices to use to sweeten what we eat. Remember the goal here is for you to have more energy. With that being said, the old adage of everything in moderation seems to apply the best. Do the research. Decide if you are okay using honey, stevia, or agave instead of sugar. Maybe you prefer adding some fresh fruit to foods to add sweetness.

Whatever you decide, do any of it in moderation. Bottom line is that with less sugar in your diet, you will have less blood sugar spikes throughout your day which in turn will lead to more energy throughout your day.

Don't Be Fooled By the Fake Stuff

While you are learning to read labels, take a little time to learn about all the different names that artificial sweeteners use. The pink, blue, or yellow packages are tempting to use on a daily basis. If you are a diabetic, it is a little more understandable. If you aren't, you really need to rethink what you are consuming.

Your body has no idea what these chemicals are — being that there are no nutrients in them. Your body has to work a lot harder at figuring out how to break them down and eliminate them from the body because they don't have any nutrients in them. If the main source of your sweetened foods comes from artificial sweeteners like aspartame, Splenda, or one of the others, consider daily how you can begin to decrease what you are consuming. Less of the fake sugar is as important for increased energy as consuming less real sugar.

Food Swaps

Once you know how much sugar you consume and where in your diet it is hiding, you now can get creative when it comes to what you eat. Instead of the yogurt with all the extra sugar or artificial sweeteners, swap it for plain yogurt with some fresh fruit added. Instead of the donut, swap it for a protein bar with low sugar and high protein and fiber. Instead of the iced latte with vanilla syrup, choose a plain iced coffee and add a little stevia and cream.

There are tons of books with alternative recipes and lots of websites with good ideas to make this process easier. Baby steps are the key here. Make little changes every day and before you know it, you will be consuming less and less sugar on a daily basis and you won't even miss it.

Synergistic effects of not giving in to your sugar cravings:

- Reduces the inflammation in your body
- Helps maintain more stable blood sugar levels
- Helps decrease tooth decay
- Helps reduce chances of more belly fat
- Decreases risk for diabetes
- Helps support a strong immune system
- Promotes a healthy digestive tract
- Decreases pain in the body
- Improves concentration
- Decreases risk for cancer
- Decreases risk for heart disease

Skipping Meals

The real reason we are supposed to eat daily is to give our bodies fuel to function. If you get too busy and forget to consume meals or just skip them thinking you want to save the calories, your body won't have the fuel that it needs to keep you functioning at an optimum level. If you want more energy evenly throughout your day, skipping meals is not an option. Eating consistent meals helps to keep your blood sugar levels stabilized so that you don't have spikes and dips in your levels during the day.

Your daily goal is to have 3 regular meals: breakfast, lunch, and dinner, as well as 2 snacks: one mid morning and one mid to late afternoon. Plan on trying to eat breakfast within one hour of rising, and then eat the remaining snacks and meals spread out over the rest of your day – approximately every 2 ½ to 3 hours.

Start With the 3 Main Meals

If you are not used to eating breakfast, lunch, and dinner, start here. Whatever meal you are missing out on daily, work on that. If breakfast is your missed meal, have a protein bar or a smoothie if time is an issue. If lunch is your missed meal, pack a lunch and take it with you so you have no excuse for not eating. If dinner is your main missed meal, plan a menu at the beginning of the week. Make sure you have all the ingredients in the house and even do a little prep work so you won't have an excuse for not cooking when you get home.

The main focus here is to make sure you get yourself in the habit of eating three main meals each day. After planning and consuming three meals per day becomes a habit, then you can look at the quality of those meals for added energy.

Add In 2 Snacks Per Day

Having a mid morning and a mid to late afternoon snack will keep your blood sugar more balanced throughout your entire day, will help increase your metabolism, and will also help to keep you from over indulging at lunch or dinner because you won't feel so overly hungry when it is mealtime. Try to choose snacks that have a good amount of protein in them so that you will stay satisfied longer. Plan out your snacks ahead of time each week and carry them with you daily so you won't be inclined to skip this important ritual.

Establish Set Meal and Snack Times

Plan a schedule for best times to eat your meals and snacks. You might vary from this schedule occasionally if a special occasion or situation comes up, but for the most part, try to have consistent times daily to eat. This will help you to be more successful at not skipping meals.

Have a Back-Up Plan

If you aren't good at cooking or preparing your lunch and snacks in advance to carry with you, you can always buy them. This will definitely be better than not eating. Do some research on the take-out restaurants in the vicinity of your job or your home. Make sure you read the labels on the meals they serve so you can make healthier choices when you are in a hurry. Have a few standard meals or snacks in mind before you go to buy anything so you will make a better choice. For example, getting a salad with grilled chicken and the dressing on the side will be a fairly safe choice almost anywhere you go. Remember, the key here is to gain more energy — not lose energy because you decided to grab a donut for a snack because you didn't have a better idea in mind before you saw it sitting in the window.

Cook In Bulk

If you do cook, think in advance. Cook meals in larger quantities so you will have leftovers. You can eat them for dinner again or even take them for your lunch. Another option is to spend some of your time on your days off preparing a few meals for the upcoming week. Once they are prepared you can freeze them for one of the nights you don't have the time or desire to cook.

Synergistic effects of not skipping meals:

- May help maintain better weight control
- Improves concentration
- Helps maintain more stable blood sugar levels
- Improves control of overeating
- Improves sleep
- Aids in less hot flashes
- Reduces risk for diabetes
- Reduces risk for heart disease

Habit *Six*

Not Drinking Enough Water

It's so easy to let the busyness of your day keep you from drinking adequate amounts of water. Most of us are in the habit of grabbing something to drink when we feel thirsty. What you might not realize is that if you become too dehydrated, your *thirst* mechanism shuts off and you won't get that thirsty cue to drink more water.

Your body needs adequate amounts of water to help flush toxins out of vital organs, to keep your ears, nose, and throat tissues moist, to carry nutrients to your cells, and to maintain body temperature. Even allowing your body to become mildly dehydrated can drain your energy, cause headaches, lightheadedness, and sleepiness.

Your body loses water daily through your breath, perspiration, urine, and bowel movements. You also need to consume more water when: you exercise or do any activity that makes you sweat; you live in a hot or humid climate; you live in or visit a higher altitude; you are battling some illnesses; and when you are a women who is breastfeeding her child.

Paying attention to how much water you consume daily is key to staying adequately hydrated because it is important that your water intake be in-line with your daily water loss.

Water is obviously the best choice for hydrating your body, but foods with high water content, like most fruits and vegetables, also count toward about 20% of your fluid intake as well as do other beverages you drink. Keep in mind though, that all beverages are not created equal, and water will always be the best fluid to ward off low energy.

If you consume at least 8 glasses a day, or close to half your body weight in ounces, you should be within a good daily range of water intake. Keep in mind that you should always drink more water before and after exercise. And if you have a job where you work outside, you may also need to consume more water — especially in the summer months.

(**Note:** if you have any special health concerns and aren't sure how much water intake is appropriate, it is important for you to consult with your healthcare provider to determine what your specific daily fluid needs are. Some health issues actually require some people to closely monitor their daily fluid intake.)

Count Your Glasses

Spend a few days keeping track of how much water and other fluids you are actually consuming. Write it down every time you drink another glass of water. Keep track at home and at work. Make sure you know how many ounces of water your favorite glass or container holds. Get a measuring cup out, fill it with water, and pour it into your drinking cup so you know for sure how many ounces it holds. Remember that one cup is equal to 8 ounces.

With the goal being at least 8 cups per day, that converts to 64 ounces of fluid daily. Don't forget to include other fluids you consume like: the milk you poured over your cereal, the coffee you purchased on your way to work, or the soda you drank with your lunch. Count everything.

Once you have figured out how much you really drink daily, you will know if this is a habit you need to work on. If you aren't drinking enough, figure out how much more you need to make your daily goal, and make sure you fill your drinking container up the appropriate amount of times daily to meet your goal.

Commit to a 21 day trial of drinking more water daily and check in with yourself every few days to evaluate how your body is feeling with regards to your energy level.

Start Your Day Off Right

Realize that when you rise in the morning, you are probably starting off a little low on fluid due to no consumption for several hours. Begin your day by drinking at least 2 full glasses of water. If you take medication in the morning, and it needs to be consumed with water, drink an entire glass at that time if the instructions don't say otherwise. If you take vitamins in the morning, drink an entire glass at that time with those as well.

Carry Water with You

If you have water with you in your car or on your desk at work, you will be more likely to remember to drink throughout the day. This is not a habit that everyone has, so you may have to figure out little tricks to remind yourself not to forget to take the water or container with you. A sticky note on the door you will see when you leave the house will help. A reminder on your car visor or even a reminder on your computer at work to drink more is another way to help yourself remember. You can even set an alarm on your phone to go off every hour. The key here is to be consistent and make it a new habit.

Add Flavor to Your Water

Water is really the best thing for your body to help with your energy. If you really want something more flavorful, try adding a slice of lemon, lime, cucumber, or even a little fresh fruit. You can actually have a pitcher of water in the fridge that you add the slices to so it becomes infused and then pour water out of the pitcher into your drinking cup.

Counter The Dehydrating Effects

Caffeinated beverages do count toward your total fluid intake even though they might not be the best choices to keep your energy level stable. Because they work in the body like a diuretic, causing the body to urinate more, you should consider drinking extra water if and when you drink more than a few cups of coffee, tea, soda, or other caffeinated beverages in one day. This will insure that your body doesn't become dehydrated.

Synergistic effects of having a body that is well hydrated:

- Improves mental speed
- Increases toxin removal from your body
- Improves hydration of skin
- Decreases joint pain
- Decreases headaches
- Decreases risk for cancer
- May help with weight loss
- Helps increase the energy in your muscles
- Helps reduce constipation
- Improves ability to exercise

Habit *Seven*_____

Trading Sleep
For Awake Time

M ost everyone does this from time to time. There happens to be a special television show on during the week that you decide to stay up late to watch. You get busy surfing on the internet and lose track of time. You need to finish just one more load of laundry before you go to bed. And the list goes on. What you stay up late to do might change daily or weekly, but that alarm clock still goes off at the same time every morning. You tell yourself you will get in bed on time and before you know it, you're hitting that snooze button in the morning and wishing you had went to bed earlier.

Your body can handle a little less sleep occasionally, but if you rob your sleep time for your awake time too often, your body will pay a huge price. Sleep is not a luxury, it's a necessity. It's as important to your overall wellness as good nutrition and exercise.

If you feel tired on a regular basis, you should not allow yourself to think that is a normal way to feel. If you are on the fence as to which habit to change first to help with your daily energy, trading sleep for awake time should definitely be your priority.

It's important to understand what happens to your body during rest. Sleep allows your body to maintain many vital functions including providing tissues and cells the opportunity to recover from the daily wear and tear of life. This is the time when your body heals and repairs your blood vessels and heart. Your immune system builds its' forces at this time.

While you sleep, your brain prepares for the next day by forming new pathways to help you remember and learn new information. Sleep helps you focus, make better life decisions, problem solve, have better coordination, control your emotions, and be creative.

Sleep deficiency has been linked to risk-taking behavior, depression, and suicide. Sleep deprivation is a risk factor for heart disease, diabetes, and obesity. You can take an occasional nap to help with how you feel, but getting a good continuous amount of sleep during the night is the only way your body will be able to repair and restore itself.

Most statistics say that adults need between 7 and 8 hours of sleep per night. The exact hours of sleep that you need will be completely individual. You might even need more than 8. You will have to look at what functions you need to do daily and whether you feel like you are performing them to the best of your ability. If you aren't, you might need to look at the possibility that you need more sleep than you are currently getting.

Start a Sleep Journal

Spend a week or two writing down everything with regards to your sleep each night. Keep track of the number of hours you sleep each night, how rested you feel the next day, how alert you feel, and how sleepy you feel. Notice if you are clumsy, short tempered, able to focus or concentrate well, and whether you are able to remember and learn things easily.

Keep track of whether you exercised the day before and at what time. Write down everything you ate and drank after 3:00 pm as well as the activities that you did in the evening hours before you went to bed. Even make a note if you woke up during the night to go to the bathroom or for some other reason. Make a note of any regular medications you might have taken as well as something extra like a cold medicine or pain reliever. If you sleep with someone, ask them if you snored or made any noises or movements in your sleep.

Once you have a good record of your sleep, you will know what you need to work on. You may need to modify how you are eating in the evening. You may need to work on your bedtime ritual or even stop taking those late naps. You may just need to go to bed earlier. You can continue trying new ways to get more restful sleep until you find the right combination of things that work best for you.

Steal Your Sleep Time Back

If you know that you need another hour or two of sleep each night, it's time to set an intention to make this a priority in your life. Figure out what you can move around in your daily schedule so that you can get that time back. You probably can't go into work later, but if that is an option, start there.

If you want to stay up to watch a television show, that is okay if you only do it one night a week. But if you are doing it every night, you are going to have to start recording the shows or opt out of watching them altogether. If you are working on homework or work until late in the evening, figure out where else in your day you can move those projects. If you are spending part of the time doing laundry, figure out a way to do it on your days off or when you first get home from work.

No matter what, if time is your issue, there are always ways to work it out if you decide to finally make this a priority.

Know What Disrupts Sleep

Heavy meals eaten less than three hours before you go to bed may cause some kind of discomfort including gas, heartburn, or bloating. Caffeine (including coffee, tea, energy drinks, soda, and chocolate) can take between 6 and 8 hours to begin to wear off. Depending upon how sensitive you are to caffeine, you should stop drinking it several hours before you go to bed.

Alcohol drank too late in the evening disrupts REM sleep and only allows lighter stages of sleep. Once it wears off, it may wake you up. Consuming some kind of nicotine product too close to bedtime also causes lighter sleep. Heavy smokers have a tendency to wake up sooner due to nicotine withdrawals.

Some medications can keep you awake or disturb your sleep. Speak with your healthcare provider or pharmacist if you think this may be an issue for you. Some women dealing with hormone fluctuations like PMS, peri-menopause, or menopause may have disrupted sleep due to hot flashes or night sweats.

Exercise is great and can help with sleep, but make sure you finish exercising at least three or more hours before you plan to go to bed. The body starts its cooling off process a few hours before you go to sleep and exercise can interfere with this process.

Short naps can be helpful at times, but make sure you don't take a nap after 3:00 pm or it may interfere with your sleep in a negative way. Keep your naps to no longer than 30 minutes.

Preparing For Sleep

For you to be able to sleep at night you have to prepare your body and your sleeping environment. Your sleeping space needs to be quiet, dark, and cool. If you have added light from a computer or other electronic devise, you may want to turn it off or move it so you can't see it from your bed.

Do some relaxing things in the evening that lets your body know it is almost bedtime—take a bath or shower, read, play soothing music, possibly dim your lights, and even consider turning off your television, computer, and cell phone. You can try different things to see what works best for you. The most important thing is to find ways to disconnect from work and the stresses of your day so that you can give your body some time to wind down and relax before you try to go to bed.

Nothing Seems To Be Working

If you have tried all of the suggestions above and you still can't consistently get good sleep at night, it may be time to have a talk with your healthcare provider. There is a possibility you suffer from some kind of sleep disorder.

The most common kinds of sleep problems/disorders are insomnia, sleep apnea, restless leg syndrome, and narcolepsy. Other health issues such as GERD and snoring can lead to these sleep disorders as well. You can use the journal notes that you prepared when you started your sleep evaluation process to show your healthcare provider.

Your healthcare provider may decide to do other blood and medical tests to rule out the possibility of you having some other health condition. They may also decide to send you to get a sleep study done to rule out some of the sleep disorders.

Synergistic effects of not trading your sleep for awake time:

- Decreases risk for obesity
- Decreases risk for diabetes
- Reduces risk for cardiovascular disease
- Increases ability to focus
- Improves problem solving skills
- Improves moodiness
- Increases ability to learn
- Improves balance and coordination
- Helps maintain a strong immune system
- Improves blood pressure
- Improves decision-making skills
- Decreases depression
- Improves memory

Not Making Physical Activity A Priority

We all know that we need to be active. No one needs to tell us this. The unfortunate thing is that since we all lead such busy lives, if you don't make a really huge effort on this one, it tends to be neglected. The other unfortunate thing is that so many people really don't like to exercise.

If you are serious about wanting to have more energy and feel your best as often as possible, you need to look into ways to make this habit a thing of the past. If you are one of those people who don't like to exercise or feel there is no way to fit it into your busy schedule, it's time to start looking at exercise in a different way.
For your body to benefit, your activity doesn't have to come from an hour workout at the gym or even a three mile daily jog in the park. There are so many ways for

you to sneak exercise into your daily routine that you might not be thinking about.

It's time to stop thinking about how you don't have enough time in your daily schedule to fit exercise in. It's time to stop focusing on how much you hate exercising. Instead, it's time to get creative and challenge yourself to figuring out new ways to fit in a little more physical activity.

Evaluate Where You Are

If you want to have more daily energy, it is time you take a serious look at what activity you do on a consistent basis. Pay attention to what you do daily and make a list. What do you do in the morning before you leave for work? Clean house, garden, walk the dog? What activity do you do at work? Do you walk a lot in your building or climb stairs? What activity do you do after work? Do you walk the dog, clean house, garden, play with the kids?

Maybe you are a stay at home mom, retired, or a student. Whatever your daily activity is, make note of it. The whole process of changing a habit starts with really evaluating what you currently do. Sometimes we get so busy living that we don't really pay attention to details of what we really do each day—it's sometimes just automatic. Once you know what activity you do regularly, then you will be able to decide how much more you really need to add.

(**Note:** If you currently have any health issues, make sure that before you add any new activities to your current routine that you speak to your healthcare provider and confirm with them that it is okay.)

Track Your Steps

One of the easiest ways to know how much movement you are getting on a daily basis is to track the steps you make daily. Wearing a pedometer is a great way to keep track of how many steps you take a day. You can use the traditional ones that clip onto your waist band or belt or you can buy ones that fit around your wrist like a watch band.

There are also apps that you can get for your phone that can help you keep track. **Fitbit fitness tracker** was one of the first fitness devices on the market to sync wirelessly to a computer. It now even syncs to your phone. It helps you keep track of your activity, exercise, weight, food and even your sleep. It helps you stay motivated by sending you a monthly report of your activity and your friends and family can be linked to your account so that you can challenge one another and keep track of who is the most active. If you are competitive, this can be a way for you to stay more motivated and you can make it more of a game than a chore.

Pedometers are a great way to see how active you really are. If you aren't as active as you thought you were, you can easily set an intention to be even more active. For example, if you currently walk 5000 steps per day, you might set an intention for yourself to increase your steps by 100 daily until you reach a goal of 1000 extra steps per day. You could stay at this level for a week or so and see how you feel.

Once you feel comfortable at that level, you might increase it by another 1000 steps. You can add extra steps to your day very easily if you put some extra thought into it. Take the stairs instead of the elevator every time you can. Whenever you go somewhere park farther from the door so you can get a few extra steps in. Take your dog for a walk — this way you both get exercise. When you go golfing, skip the golf cart. When you go to the post office to mail a letter, park your car and walk inside instead of driving by the box. Take a five or ten minute walk on your lunch hour.

It doesn't matter what you do, what matters is the fact that your mind is thinking about what unique ways you can incorporate into your daily activity so that you can get in just a few more steps.

If your intention was to walk 7,000 steps for the day, and toward the end of the day you find yourself short of that goal by 100 steps, consider creating and walking a course inside your house. It could be around the living room or around the kitchen table. Any open area in the house or even in the garage will work. Once you do a few laps, you will find that you easily made it to your goal of 7,000 steps. This is a great way to get your steps in when the weather is bad and you can't go outside.

Obviously, you could accomplish the same thing on a treadmill, but not everyone has access to one, and for some, using a treadmill might feel more like you're exercising than just walking around the house. This process is all about you figuring out what works for you and helps you to stick with an exercise plan. Before you know it, it might even feel like a game and not exercise at all.

Exercise in Intervals

Studies have shown that whether you exercise for a full 30 minutes or break that time up into 10 minute intervals three times during your day, you still get great health benefits. Many people don't feel like they can find the time to exercise for 30 minutes straight. But if you change your thinking and get a little creative, you can easily find 10 minutes to exercise three times per day.

If you can sneak the first 10 minutes in before your morning shower, you will find it starts your day off with more energy. Some ideas of how to get in 10 minutes of exercising before work: walk your dog, vacuum your house, hold a few yoga poses, walk your house stairs, or even walk a few laps around the living room and kitchen.

To get in 10 minutes of exercise in the middle of your work day, try: walking the stairs at work, do some stretches or yoga poses in the bathroom, walk in the parking lot on your break or lunch hour, grab a co-worker and walk somewhere close by for lunch.

If you aren't working, instead of meeting for coffee or lunch, meet a friend for an activity like golf, hiking, or a dance class. Go shopping and walk around the mall a few times before actually going into any of the stores.

In the evening, get 10 minutes of exercise in by: walking around your neighborhood, lifting small weights or jumping rope while you wait for your dinner to cook; stretching or doing leg lifts while watching the news or during television commercials; playing a game of basketball or tag with your kids; or even trimming a few rose bushes or weeding a flower bed.

Any activity that gets your heart rate elevated and gets you using different muscle groups in your body for at least 10 minutes will be so much more beneficial for you then plopping down in front of the television or computer screen and being idle for hours at a time.

On your days off, consider saving money on a gardener and choose to mow, rake, and trim your own yard. When looking for activities to do with your family, skip the movies or dinner and go to the zoo or a local museum, ride your bikes, or walk the trails in a local park. Skip the car wash and hand wash your car. Take a class and learn something new like yoga, swing dancing, tai chi, or kayaking. Choose to hand wash the windows inside and outside your house instead of paying someone else to do the job for you. Grab a group of friends and go dancing for the evening instead of going out to eat dinner.

Any activity that gets you moving, works different muscle groups, and raises your heart rate will be beneficial to your body and your energy level. Instead of thinking about how much you don't like exercising, think instead about how you can combine exercise with your workday, housework, and after work activities so that it doesn't feel like you just worked out.

Challenge yourself to thinking about creative ways to combine activity with your daily duties and you will be reaping the benefits of extra energy before you know it.

Synergistic effects of getting more physical activity:

- Aids in ability to be more alert
- Helps increase your metabolism
- Improves blood pressure
- Helps improve productivity at work
- Increases your longevity
- Helps reduce falls for older adults
- May help maintain better weight control
- Reduces risk for cardiovascular disease
- Reduces risk for diabetes
- May help strengthen muscles and bones
- Improves mood
- Helps decrease stress
- Improves relationships
- Decreases depression
- Improves coordination

Part 3

Emotional Health Habits

Habit *Nine*_____

Not Scheduling Down Time For Yourself

Over working and over committing can be physically and mentally draining. It can lead to poor health, a poor ability to focus, a decrease in problem solving abilities, a decrease in creative flow, and the list goes on. To keep up with the stress of a busy life, you must learn to make self-care a priority. If you think of self-care as a luxury, it's time to change your thinking. It's an absolute necessity if you want to have a life with more energy.

Contrary to how society makes us feel sometimes about taking care of ourselves, self-care is not self-indulgent. Self-care is the best way to help your body rest and recharge when you begin to feel emotionally or physically drained. It is not really as much about what you choose to do as it is about making sure you do something to re-charge your battery.

Some days it's about having some time to not have to think or *be on*. It doesn't matter whether you are a man or a woman, the need is the same. Choosing to take some down time to care for ourselves means we will be *more on* and *more available* for anyone we interact with or care for.

Evaluate Your Self-Care Practice

Spend some time thinking about this. Step back and be objective. If you aren't sure you are being objective, ask a close friend or relative to help you decide. Make a list of what things you do that you feel are part of a self-care practice. Make a note of how often you do those things for yourself. Some examples might be: taking a hot bath, watching a sporting event, getting a manicure, getting a massage, taking a nap, working in your garden, watching a movie, reading a book, or going dancing.

What you do with the time you set aside for yourself is not important. What is important is that you do something that brings you joy and recharges you.

Once you have a list of what you currently do for yourself, take a little time to think about how you feel you are handling stress in your life. Decide if your daily or weekly self-care routine is helping to keep your stress at bay. If it isn't, you know you need to find a way to add more self-care time into your schedule. There are a lot of ways to help manage your stress — self-care is an important one and should never be negotiable.

Schedule It

If you lead a crazy, busy life, the best way for you to have time for your self-care might just be to actually schedule it on your calendar. If you do have to do this, make sure you treat the time as if it were a work project. For instance, if you want to use your self-care time to go and watch the ducks in the park, make sure you block out enough time in your schedule for driving to and from as well as a good amount of time to relax and watch the ducks. Treat this time just like you would any other important commitment. Remind yourself that time you schedule for yourself is important — it helps to keep you on track, have less stress, and in the end, more energy as well.

Be Careful About Swapping

You may occasionally be tempted to swap one self-care time and day for another or even completely give it up. Sometimes important work projects come up or family issues need to be taken care of and we have no choice but to put ourselves and priorities on hold. This is how life rolls sometimes.

The key here is to not allow yourself to get into a habit of letting your self-care always take a back seat to everything and everyone else. It's okay to swap days or times occasionally, but if you see a pattern starting, fight yourself to get back on track. You matter. The time you spend recharging is extremely important to helping you manage your stress so you can be at your best every day.

Never Feel Guilty

No matter what, never allow yourself to feel guilty because you take time to take care of yourself. Guilt is your friend. Never allow yourself to feel like spending time on yourself could be better spend by finishing just one more project at work or one more chore at home. Remind yourself that by doing something for yourself, you will have the energy and focus you need to finish that work project and do more chores at home.

It's Okay To Add More Time

This book is all about you learning to slow down and listen to your body. If you don't, how will you know what needs to change so you can have better days. If you realize at any point that you don't feel like you are spending enough time re-charging, step back and do another evaluation of your situation.

Have you given up some of your self-care time to finish a project or attend to a family commitment? Has your work load been busier than usual lately? If either of these are the case, maybe you need to work on your schedule and find a way to add more time in for yourself. Maybe you will only need to do it for a week or two and maybe this is a sign that you just haven't been doing enough. Whatever the case, it's important that you find a way to make more time for yourself.

The beauty of learning to listen to your body is being able to tweak things up when life throws you a few curve balls.

Combining Priorities

If you really feel crunched for time, you could occasionally consider combining some of your self-care routine with other life responsibilities. Don't make this a habit because you do need some quiet, alone time on a regular basis, but occasionally this is okay. An example of this might be that you committed to taking your son to soccer practice and the day got changed to a day you had planned to spend some down time reading a new novel you had bought. You could still take him to the practice and instead of talking to the other parents or watching him practice, you could find yourself a place to yourself and start reading your novel. Not the most optimum, but still helpful for your overall ability to re-boot. You may lose part of your time, but at least you won't feel completely deprived.

Synergistic effects of building more down time into your schedule:

- Helps maintain a strong immune system
- Increases positive thinking
- Promotes a sense of being more calm
- Increases body's ability to adapt to stress
- Decreases depression
- Increases creativity
- Increases emotional wellbeing
- Improves sleep
- Increases self-esteem
- Improves ability to exercise
- Improves relationships
- Aids in ability to be a better caretaker

Lacking Daily Interactions With Uplifting People

Having daily interactions with other people is food for the soul. It helps you stay positive and feel like you aren't alone in the world. It also helps you to feel more connected to others and not so isolated. As humans we are wired to make connections with other humans. It's not only important to have interactions with other people on a daily basis, but it is just as important to have those connections be with uplifting people—people who are positive, supportive, and have similar likes and dislikes as yourself.

If you want your energy level to continue moving in a positive direction, it's time you take a serious look at the people you spend time with on a daily basis.

Evaluate Your Relationships

Spend some quiet time making a list of everyone that you consistently spend time with. Next to each person's name, write down whether you think that person gives you energy, or takes your energy away. Also, make a note of what common interests you share with each person on your list.

Once you have a completed list of your relationships, you can begin to look at which ones serve you well and bring joy to your life, and which ones zap your energy and bring more frustration to your life. Spend a week or two really paying attention to how you feel after you spend time with each of the people on your list. Do you feel a negative vibe or a decrease in your energy levels? Do you find yourself feeling less confident in yourself, or partaking in more negative self-talk when you spend time with some people? Is it only occasionally or is it every time you interact with them?

This can be a hard habit to work on because sometimes we don't feel like we have a choice whom we spend our time with. But you really do. It's time to be honest with yourself and make a serious effort to work on this area of your life if you truly want to have more energy on a daily basis.

Spend Your Time Wisely

Once you have evaluated your relationships, the next part of the process is really pretty simple. Spend more time with the people who give you energy and less time, or no time, with the people who zap your energy. If any of the energy zappers are family members or co-workers, you will have to be creative in how you choose to decrease the time you spend with them.

For family, it might be about staying on topics of conversation that relate to something important to both of you whether that be regarding family, or a common interest. Once the topic of conversation goes in a negative direction, have an escape plan in place and get away from them as soon as possible. As for a co-worker, keep your interactions with them specifically tied to work related things. Find a way to politely excuse yourself when you feel the conversation is going in a negative direction and say you have a project to complete or a phone call you forgot you needed to make.

Meet New People

If you don't have any quality relationships in your life, or you only have a few, it is definitely time to start finding new ways to meet new people. For some people this is pretty easy. For others it can be more of a challenge. Don't let fear of the unknown get in your way. Ask other positive people you know to introduce you to some of their friends and acquaintances. Go to events, gatherings, or classes that attract other like minded people who share in a common interest. While you are on a lunch break at work, strike up a conversation with the new employee—you never know whether you might share some similar interests.

Remember that you may only have a few things in common with some people. But that's okay. The most important thing is that you feel energized when you spend time with them. You may have one friend that enjoys going to the theater with you while on the other hand you have a completely different friend who hates the theater, but loves to play golf like you do. As long as you have a few things in common and you feel energized while you are with them, that's all that matters.

Get Out Of the House

If you are in a place in your life where you realize you are a little on the lonely side, but aren't feeling confident enough to build new relationships, commit yourself to making a daily effort to get out of the house. Loneliness is normal and is a signal that it is time for you to get yourself motivated to get out and seek new relationships. If you are going through some kind of life transition—a divorce, loss of a loved one, retirement, or maybe you made a recent move to a new city—whatever the case, it is really important that you don't allow yourself to sit at home and spend all of your down time by yourself. Loneliness and isolation can lead to other health issues besides just low energy.

Make small trips out of the house daily. Strike up small conversations with people who work in the stores you go to—for example in a bookstore, library, or hobby store. Go out to a small coffee shop or restaurant where there are lots of people enjoying themselves. Strike up a conversation with someone sitting near you. If you are in a new school, look for a club to join that interests you. If you are on a new job, find out if there is a common place the staff goes together on their off time and ask if you can join. If you are in a new neighborhood, strike up a conversation with a neighbor while you take a walk around the block. It doesn't matter what you do, just interact with other people daily.

Consider Therapy

If you find that you aren't able to meet new people and build positive relationships, it may be time to consider finding a therapist to work with. Therapy can help you hone your skills and approaches to relationships. A good therapist can help you gain new insight into yourself and help you build confidence to go out into the world with a new outlook and approach to life and relationships.

Synergistic effects of having daily interactions with uplifting people:

- Improves overall feeling of wellbeing
- Improves loneliness
- Improves depression
- Improves ability to exercise
- Improves longevity
- Improves blood pressure
- Supports immune health
- Helps reduce chances of obesity
- Decreases addictive behavior
- Improves sleep

Habit *Eleven*

Not Listening To Your Life's Calling

A lot of us cling to a job that is a bad fit. There is a voice deep inside of us that tries to speak out, but often we hush it up and tell it to mind its own business. Life is stressful enough already. Doing something risky will only create more chaos and anxiety in our overcomplicated lives. That crazy voice needs to be ignored. Right?

Wrong! For us to thrive without anxiety, it is an inner necessity for us to figure out our life's work. To feel joy, fulfillment, and daily energy, you have to be living your authentic life as your authentic self. It's not about conforming to an image of what others think you should be. It's about learning to listen to your inner voice. It's about learning to trust what you cannot see.

We all need to figure out what our unique part in the world is — the part that is individual to each of us.

You were put here on this earth for a reason. It's time for you to quit ignoring that inner voice and get down to business. The business of figuring out how you can live your authentic life and be a person filled with a zest for life on a mission to follow the path of your authentic vocation.

Evaluate Where You Are

Believe it or not, this will probably be the easiest part of the process. If you don't feel like you are doing work that fulfills you, admit it to yourself. It doesn't matter if it is the only work you have ever done in your work career. It doesn't matter if you went to school for four years or ten years. It doesn't matter if your family thinks this is what you were meant to do. It doesn't even matter if originally it was what you thought you should do or wanted to do.

What matters is whether your soul is crying out for a change. What matters is whether you wake up daily with a funny feeling in the pit of your stomach because you realize it is time to get up and go to work — a work you really have no real desire to do. What matters is whether *you* are happy with *your* life.

How you go about evaluating where you are is a completely individual process. The whole process of finding your life's purpose is completely individual.

Some people meditate on a regular basis and feel this brings them clarity on what to do in their life. If this isn't already part of your daily routine, this is definitely a place to start. (Read the section in this book titled, "Not Taking Time Daily to Quiet Your Mind.")

Part of the evaluation process should be about looking back and seeing the signs that have been screaming at you over the years to take notice of your dissatisfying life. Write down every major incident that stands out over the past 10 or 20 years that you think shows that you weren't happy with your life and then write out which incidences showed that you were incredibly happy. Pay close attention to everything — things that had to do with jobs and things that had to do with personal events or even hobbies that you did. Try to determine why some things made you happy and other things didn't.

Make sure that you include information about your current job as well. What parts of it bring you joy, and what parts do you dread doing?

There is no right or wrong way to do this. This is about you learning to listen to your soul and you learning to be completely honest with yourself. More than likely, this process will be incredibly uncomfortable and it may even be downright painful. But evaluating what isn't working for you with regards to your current career is absolutely necessary if you want to get to the heart of your true calling.

Figure Out What Brings You Pleasure

Keep your list of what things have brought you joy over the past 10 or 20 years close by. Refer back to it as you go through this next process. It's time to go on a treasure hunt. Spend at least a month or two doing this process. You can spend longer if you find it necessary.

Your mission is to get a notebook and start writing down every person, place, or thing that brings great joy to your life. These may be things you come in contact with while you are doing your normal everyday business and they can be things or people you actually go out of your way to connect with.

Keep your notebook with you at all times. Be on high alert. Whatever you see that interests you, whomever you meet that brings a smile to your face, whatever you do that feels right, take note of it. It's okay to go out of your way some days to see new things, meet new people, and do new things. If you are reading the newspaper and you see information about an event that sounds intriguing, make plans to go. If a friend needs a volunteer to help with a charity event, be the volunteer. If you see a sign advertising a new business, do an internet search if it peaks your interest.

Nothing is off limits. Give yourself permission to get off track and waste time. This is your life's mission. You can only figure out what your life's calling is by living your life to the fullest and taking notice of what brings you great joy.

Stop Thinking and Start Surrendering

If you want to begin the process of figuring out what your purpose in life is, you can no longer continually push through life, keep a crazy busy schedule, and ignore your inner voice. You have to stop your own ego's voice from being the most predominate voice in your head and instead begin allowing your soul's voice to be the one that shines through. Your ego wants you to do a lot of thinking; your soul wants you to do a lot of feeling.

If you want to find your true calling, it's time to surrender to your soul. It is time to learn to trust what you cannot see. It might be challenging at first to learn to trust your inner voice, but with practice, you will find that it will get easier.

Work Backwards

As you go through this process of listening to your soul, you are slowly learning who you don't want to be when you grow up. That's a powerful thing to know. Knowing what you aren't interested in and knowing what doesn't feed your soul, helps you to get closer to your life's calling. Don't allow yourself to look at not finding your way as a mistake—look at it as being one step closer to figuring out what your authentic life looks like. Be kind to yourself. This is not a black and white process. You can only know what you do want by figuring out what you don't want.

Stop Listening to Other People

It isn't about what anyone else thinks you should be or do. No one can truly know but you. People usually mean well, but their own personal fear and lack of confidence in themselves is usually what causes them to be a naysayer and question your intentions. You need to speak up and tell them that the best way they can help you is not by interjecting their opinions, but by providing support for where you currently are.

It's important that you don't allow anyone else to shake the confidence you have in your abilities to listen to your inner voice.

It's Okay to Change Your Mind

Since part of this process is figuring out what doesn't feed your soul, you may find yourself changing your mind a lot. Don't allow yourself to be crippled by this process. Sometimes you will just know before you try something new that it isn't the right direction for you. And sometimes, you may have to get into the middle of something, before you realize that it's all wrong. Part of the reason this happens is because we allow our ego to take charge again, we think too much, and before we know it, we have lost touch with our inner voice again. This is like falling off a bike. Don't let a skinned knee get you down. Get back up and keep going.

Stop Being Who You Aren't

If you want this process to work, you have to be honest with yourself. It is a universal tendency to want to be someone else, but in the end, you need to be yourself. This process will be painful at times as you figure out who you aren't supposed to be and wish you knew exactly who you should be. Surrender any and all notions, trust your inner guidance system, make peace with who you aren't supposed to be, and stop being who you aren't supposed to be. Because if you don't stop being who you aren't supposed to be, how will you ever be who you were meant to be.

Synergistic effects of listening to your life's calling:

- Aids in feeling more joy
- Helps promote a strong immune function
- Reduces risk for all major diseases
- Increases life span
- Improves daily focus
- Decreases daily stress
- Reduces the inflammatory response
- Improves coping skills
- Improves mood
- Reduces risk for obesity
- Improves sex drive
- Promotes a healthy digestive tract
- Helps reduce pain
- Improves depression

Habit **Twelve**_____

Overlooking The Fact
That You Overeat

Figuring out how to have more energy daily has everything to do with trying to balance as many aspects of your life as possible. If you occasionally or consistently find yourself overeating, you won't be able to address your low energy concerns unless you meet this habit head on. Food is supposed to be fuel for the body, but sometimes life causes us to forget that fact. Overeating can be about so much more than cravings and nutrient deficiencies in the body. It can be about: feelings of deprivation, depression, lack of willpower, boredom, anxiety, and sometimes low self-esteem.

It's important that you really pay attention to the cues your body is giving you. Are you really hungry or are you just eating because it tastes good or for emotional comfort? If you find yourself consistently overeating anything — carbohydrates, processed foods, salty items, sweets, or even entire meals — it is time you take a closer look at what is causing you to have this habit. You owe it to yourself and the future health of your body.

Evaluate Why and When You Overeat

Begin by journaling for a week or two. Keep track daily of all the food you consume. Write down what time of day you ate the food item or meal. Also make a note of how you were feeling when you ate the food item or meal. Look for patterns. Do you eat while watching television? Does a stressful day at work cause you to binge? Do you take comfort in food after an argument with your significant other? Does a walk past a full length mirror in the bedroom send you looking for that new bag of potato chips you just bought? Does most of your overeating occur while you are dining outside of your house?

Spend time deciding how you have been feeling lately. Have you felt bored, deprived, disgusted with yourself, or overwhelmed with your life? Once you recognize a pattern as to why and when you overeat, you can work on ways to overcome the urge.

Plan for What Triggers You

Depending upon what your triggers are, you can create a plan to help keep you from overindulging the next time the urge comes.

If you eat due to boredom, have some healthy snacks available (like cut up fresh vegetables) so you won't go for the bag of potato chips. If you use food as a pick-me-up for a bad mood, choose a snack that is a good mix of both protein and carbohydrates like a handful of nuts or cottage cheese and fresh fruit. Better yet, if your mood is low, maybe playing your favorite music or taking a walk in the fresh air will work just as well.

If watching television is a trigger for you, maybe you can do a few floor exercises or stretches when you get that urge to eat. If you are feeling deprived, keep some low sugar fruit popsicles in the freezer or a few pieces of low sugar hard candy so you can have a sweet treat without overindulging.

If the majority of your overeating occurs while dining outside of your house, plan ahead. If you will be going to a gathering where there are lots of snack foods available, eat a light, balanced meal before you leave home so you won't be starved when you get there. Plan on using the smallest plate possible and put only a few items on the plate so you will feel okay about going back for seconds. Drink a glass of water in between small servings.

If you go to a restaurant to dine, consider: sharing a meal with someone, ordering off the appetizer menu, or ask for a to-go box when your food arrives and box half of the meal up to take home. This way you won't be tempted to eat the whole meal in one sitting.

There are lots of ways that you can head your triggers off at the pass. Knowing what your triggers are, having a plan in place for when you find yourself in that situation, acknowledging to yourself that you are about to overeat, and then taking action to stop the process.

You have the willpower to make these changes. Just focus on one day at a time and one situation at a time. Be patient, but firm with yourself. If you do slip on any day, forgive yourself and begin again.

Work on Your Self-Care

Because so much of overeating is an emotional process, it is imperative that you make your self-care a priority. For a man, self- care might have to do with working on a special home project, spending time watching sports, reading a good book, going on a bike ride, or hanging out with the guys. For a woman, self-care might have to do with making the time to read a good book or magazine, taking a bath, getting a massage, or going shopping with friends.

It doesn't matter what activity you do—as long as you carve out some time weekly to do something that is important to you, helps keep your stress levels down, and feeds your soul.

(For more suggestions in this area, check out the section in the book titled, "Not Scheduling Down Time For Yourself.")

Seek Professional Help

If you try the suggestions above, and you still feel like your eating habits are out of control, it might be time to seek professional help. Speak with your healthcare provider and let them decide if this may be an issue that they need to run some tests for to rule out any deficiencies in your body.

Other options that you can consider are joining a special group for overeaters or seeking one-on-one counseling with someone who specializes in this professional area. If sitting in an office with a professional counselor isn't something that you think you would be comfortable with, find a professional that does counseling over the phone.

Be aware that sometimes this issue is so much bigger than one person can handle on his or her own. You deserve to have the best life possible. Look at seeking a counselor as being a form of self- care.

Synergistic effects of not overeating:

- Helps maintain more stable blood sugar levels
- Decreases brain fog
- Helps reduce cravings for poor quality foods
- Improves self-confidence
- May help maintain better weight control
- Decreases risk for chronic disease
- Improves self image

*Thirteen*_____

Disregarding Your Blue Mood

Mental battles that rage within us are just as significant as the physical problems that arise in the body. The biggest difference is that society feels more comfortable talking about physical body problems than it does mental issues. If you have lost your drive and your energy to do the most basic things in life, you may have a bigger problem than you realize. You may be suffering from depression.

Not only is it difficult for society to acknowledge how prevalent depression is, it is hard for individuals who have the issues to admit it to themselves. If you truly want to have more energy physically and emotionally, it is time you really listen closely to your body and acknowledge what it is telling you.

Keep in mind that there can be varying degrees of depression—from mild to moderate to severe. Some of the symptoms that you may be experiencing could be related to nutritional deficiencies, health conditions, or even recent or past life experiences. You may be able to help yourself by working on a more balanced meal plan, adding in some nutritional supplements, working with a counselor, or possibly taking some prescription medications.

The most important thing is that you admit to yourself that you are having signs of depression and make a conscious decision to do something about it.

Journal Your Symptoms

Spend a week or two watching how you deal with everyday life and write down what happens daily, how you respond, and how you feel about people, your job, and about life in general. Pay attention to your energy level. Take note if you over indulge in any addictive behaviors like smoking, drinking, substance use, eating, gambling, or sex.

Pay attention to whether you consistently have cravings for sugar, carbohydrates, or caffeine. Do you have rapid mood swings, are you disinterested in things you used to like to do, or do you seem more irritable at times? Do you find yourself being more negative about life, are you anxious, or do you feel like you have the blahs? Do you tend to be more sensitive to life's pain, do you have trouble concentrating, or do you find yourself venting or rehashing personal problems from the past? Do you sleep through the night and if so, do you wake feeling rested? Do you sleep too much and have trouble getting up?

It's important to also make a note of any changes that have occurred within the past year or so of your life. Have you suffered a major trauma or the loss of a loved one? Have you lost a job or retired from your job of several years? Have you had a beloved pet recently die? Did your child recently leave the nest? Maybe you had surgery and lost a body part. Maybe you were in a tragic car accident. These are all situations that can cause a person to grieve. Grief can lead to depression in some people. No two people grieve exactly the same way. Some people take much longer to get through the process than others.

You can also ask your spouse, a relative, or a close friend if they see any differences in your moods or your reactions to life situations. These are all things to take note of when you start your journaling. It is extremely important that you be honest with yourself.

Speak with an Expert

Whether you want to try to deal with this on your own, or get a professional's help, you have to know for sure what all you are dealing with. You have the ability to change up your diet and exercise plan, but you don't know for sure what might be going on chemically inside your body.

Depression can be caused by so many individual things as well as a combination of things. Seeing your healthcare provider and ruling out any major health issues can help make your process easier. Your physician can do blood tests and look for deficiencies in vitamin B and D levels as well as other nutritional levels. They can also check your thyroid, look for other hormone imbalances, and test for adrenal fatigue.

You can use your journaling record to help your healthcare provider understand how you are feeling and it can be a guide for them to decide where to start.

Once you have had a few blood tests to rule out or confirm deficiencies or hormone issues, then you can come up with a plan together with your healthcare provider to help with your depression. This might also be a good time to decide if nutritional therapy will be enough or if psychotherapy might be necessary as well.

Your healthcare provider may also suggest that you begin taking some kind of prescription pharmaceutical product. Keep in mind that there are a lot of great alternative options for depression available—you just have to be willing to do the research and find a healthcare provider that is willing to work with you to try the alternative approach.

Check out the book titled *"The Mood Cure"* by Julia Ross, M.A. It is a great resource with lots of alternative ways to help with mood disorders. There are also several good books available to help you deal with hormone issues in an alternative way if that happens to be the issue. Spend some time at your local bookstore or do some internet searches for other resources.

Raise your Serotonin Level

Serotonin is a hormone that is classified as an inhibitory neurotransmitter. It sends and transmits nerve impulses to the brain. It is found both in the brain and the digestive tract.

According to the Mayo Clinic, lower levels of serotonin in the brain can put a person at risk for developing depressive disorder. There are several things that can cause a depletion of serotonin in the body—chronic exposure to high-stress situations, lack of adequate exercise, a poor diet, lack of sufficient light, and stimulants (such as caffeine, diet pills, ephedra, and cocaine).

You can naturally raise the levels of serotonin by making a few lifestyle modifications. Soak up more sunshine during appropriate times of the year or invest in a light box to use inside your home during the winter months. Pick some kind of physical activity that you enjoy doing and make it a part of your weekly schedule. Yoga, tai chi, or qigong may be great activity choices because they can offer a stress relieving component as well as exercise.

Work on your diet. Stay away from low-calorie diets, eliminate caffeine—soda and coffee, and eliminate all artificial sweetened foods and beverages. Get in the habit of not skipping meals and eat a diet with a balance of protein, good fats, vegetables, fruits, and legumes (grains). Figure out a way that works best for you to de-stress as often as you can.

(Check out the other sections in the book titled "Skipping Meals" and "Not Scheduling Down Time for Yourself.")

Synergistic effects of treating your blue mood:

- Supports a strong immune system
- Improves sleep
- Helps maintain a positive outlook on life
- Increases ability to focus
- Increases confidence level
- Decreases risk for chronic diseases
- Helps decrease addictive behavior
- Improves ability to exercise
- Improves relationships

Overlooking the Clutter in Your Living Space

Have you ever walked into a room of your house and felt overcome by anxiety after you caught a glimpse of several piles of dirty clothes, several weeks of junk mail, or maybe even a dozen or so cook books you piled up weeks ago after looking for a recipe for your dinner? In that exact moment you once again realize that time has slipped by and you still can't check that project off of your to-do list.

No one's house can stay perfectly organized all the time—that would be an overwhelming job to keep up with. We all learn to be okay with a little untidiness now and then. But if you have large amounts of clutter in any of your living spaces, you probably walk by it daily feeling at least a little bit overwhelmed. And if you realize that the bill you need to pay is sitting somewhere deep inside the huge pile of mail on your kitchen counter, the process of finding it could be a negative pull on your energy.

If you deal with any clutter in your home or work place, it might be time for you to figure out a way to get things organized. Clutter affects us both physically and emotionally. Huge amounts of dust can collect around cluttered areas and irritate allergies, asthma, and other respiratory problems. If you have to sort through piles of things to find one item, it can take a lot of extra valuable time you usually don't have. It creates stress and embarrassment when you think about inviting people over to visit. It can cause conflicts with other family members regarding who is responsible for cleaning up problem areas.

Clutter can create anxiety and keeps you from being able to relax during your down time. Who can work on a hobby, relax and read a book, practice a few yoga poses, or feel okay inviting someone over when clutter is starring them in the face? It can also create a since of frustration because you have continued to keep something just because the item is attached to a good or bad memory, a dream, or a "someday I might need it" mentality. Some experts also believe that clutter-related stress can trigger someone to overeat—a practice that could definitely lead to obesity, lower self-esteem, and several other health problems.

You owe it to yourself to figure out a way to get your home back in order. It will be a process and you will have to be patient with yourself. It didn't get cluttered overnight so you can't expect to fix it overnight either.

The most important thing is that you recognize how important it is to work on this habit. Many areas of your life can be helped by clearing the clutter and putting together a plan to keep it from continuing to be a problem.

Evaluate Where You Have Issues

With pen and paper in hand, go from room to room in your home and make a note of what areas in each room need major attention. Make sure you don't just write down entire living room needs to be de-cluttered. Instead, write something like: bookshelf needs to be sorted, coffee table needs clearing, or area near door needs to be organized. If you break up each room into smaller sections, your sorting process won't feel so overwhelming.

Once you have been through your entire home, you now can work on a plan of how you will accomplish the tasks ahead. Remember that you aren't going to try to tackle everything at once. You are going to divide up the rooms and the sections of the rooms so you will feel like it is doable.

Pick Days and Times to Work on De-Cluttering

How much time you spend will depend upon your schedule. Initially, try working for 10 to 15 minutes at least every other day and see how that feels. If that is manageable and you feel you can do more, add a few more minutes weekly. Maybe you will decide that one or two days a week will work and you will do a bigger chunk of time on one weekend day.

It doesn't matter how you divide up your time, it just matters that you set-up a workable plan and you keep persevering. If at any time you find yourself getting stuck, take a step back, ask yourself what the issue might be and figure out a way to work around it. Some parts of the job will be more difficult than others due to the possibility of emotional attachments you might have with some of the items that you will need to sort through. Don't let it stop you, but be patient with yourself.

Set-up a System for Sorting

Gather boxes, bags, or bins to put items in as you sort. Decide how you will sort your items. Some possible choices might be: donate, trash, keep, give to a specific person, or save for garage sale. Put a label on the boxes and bins so you know what sorted items go where. If anything stumps you while you sort, and you just can't figure out what to do with a specific item, make a "not sure yet" pile and move on.

Start Small and Simple

Once you know how you will sort everything, you can begin the organization process. Don't allow yourself to think about how many rooms there are to work on. Your focus is on only one room and only one small section of that room. That's it—just one small section at a time. Once you complete one small section of a room, move onto another small section of the same room.

Stick with working on just one room at a time until you finish de-cluttering the entire room. Once one room is completed, you can then move on to a different room. By accomplishing one entire room at a time, you will feel such a sense of accomplishment that it will be your motivator to keep moving and working on more sections of your home.

If one room is too painful once you begin the process, pick another area of another room and leave the one painful room to be finished on another day. You will know when the time is right to try again. Don't beat yourself up if this does happen to you — be patient with yourself.

For piles or areas that have a lot of small items like books, mail, toys, or magazines, you may have to sort through those at a different time than larger items because they will be a little more tedious. While you are watching television is a great time to sort through a lot of small items. That way it doesn't feel as much like a chore.

Enlist the Help of Others

If you feel up to it, ask other family members or friends to help with the process. Choose someone that you feel can be objective and that will help you stay focused. There is a good possibility that you will become sentimental about some of the items that you need to get rid of so make sure that you choose someone that will help you stay on task.

Create a System for Mail

One problem so many people have an issue with is mail they receive daily. Before you tackle this problem, make sure you decide on a plan that you will follow after you clear the clutter. Whether you choose to get bins, trays, a filing cabinet, or a shredder, it doesn't really matter. You decide what might work for you and your family. Commit yourself to trying something to see if you can keep the problem under control. There are a lot of websites and books with tips on how to accomplish this. Check out some ideas before you go out and purchase any organizing systems.

If there are several people in your household, you have to decide if everyone will take a part in the new organization process or whether it will be only one person's responsibility.

You may decide to sort bills and junk mail every day when you bring the mail into the house. This way you touch it one time and it never gets out of control. If you bring mail into the house and don't sort it right away, it is highly likely that it will stay in the spot you place it and become a huge messy pile again.

If you want to keep your clutter issue from being a continued problem, you have to create some new habits going forward.

Reward Yourself

Any unwanted items that you decide to get rid of can be held and sold at a garage sale. This is a great way to make a little cash and buy yourself a reward for accomplishing your huge task. Some people work better if there is a prize at the end of the process. This can be a way of motivating you to finally finish your de-cluttering project.

Synergistic effects of not overlooking the clutter in your living space:

- Improves depression
- Improves allergies
- Improves asthma
- Improves control of overeating
- Improves ability to exercise
- Helps decrease stress levels
- Improves relationships
- Improves ability to relax at home
- Improves emotional wellbeing
- Improves immune function
- Improves air quality inside the house

Not Taking Time Daily To Quiet Your Mind

Because we expect our bodies and minds to do so much with fewer resources than ever before, meditation is a great way to relieve our daily stress so that we actually have the energy to do and be more.

Not only does meditation help reduce stress and anxiety, but it also creates an inner calm and peace within you and helps you be able to have more clarity. It can be learned by anyone, is inexpensive, and doesn't require you to purchase any special equipment.

There is no one perfect way to quiet your mind and it doesn't matter whether you practice in a formal or informal way. It is more about spending quiet time with yourself and not allowing yourself to focus on any of the jumbled thoughts inside your head.

All you really need is a few minutes of quality quiet time to meditate. As you practice more often and begin to feel the benefits, you may want to increase the time for your daily practice. You can start your day off with the process, or set an intention to find a few minutes sometime within your day.

What matters most is that you carve out regular time in your daily schedule. If you are stressed out by the thought of trying to fit this into your schedule every day, commit yourself to three days per week instead of every day. This is about you figuring out what works for you.

A lot of people try meditation once or twice and then quit. One reason so many people don't stick with meditation is because they find it difficult to focus on one thing for long periods of time. This is something everyone has trouble with. Meditation takes practice. Know that this happens to everyone, not just you.

If you are meditating to calm your mind and your attention wanders, slowly bring your attention back to the mantra, object, movement, or sensation that you were focused on. Don't allow yourself to judge your meditation skills. Judging yourself will only cause you extra stress. Also, don't allow yourself to compare how you do this process to how anyone else does it.

Know that there are a lot of different ways to quiet your mind, just like there are a lot of ways to get more energy. You may need to try more than one technique until you find what feels right for you. If one way feels really difficult for you, move on to the next way. You may decide that you actually like more than one way. If so, mix it up.

Focus On Your Breath

A lot of beginners start out using this technique. This form of meditation can be done anytime you are alone and in a quiet place. Your focus will be on feeling and listening as you inhale and exhale through your nose. If your attention wanders, slowly bring your focus back to your breathing. You can do this on your own, find a meditation CD, or take a class.

Scan Your Body

For this meditation technique, you focus on some part of your body. For example, you might start with your focus on your left foot, being aware of: any sensations, tension, pain, warmth, or relaxation within it. You then might move over to your right foot and focus your awareness on it. Slowly you will move your attention up your body from your feet, then to your ankles, and then to another new section of your body until you reach your head. This technique might also be combined with some kind of breathing exercise as well.

Repeat A Mantra

For this meditation technique you silently repeat a mantra as you meditate. A mantra is a powerful name, sound, or vibration that allows the mind to experience a deeper awareness and helps keep you focused. Repeating the mantra helps you disconnect from the thoughts crowding your mind. Mantras are generally sacred in nature. One very popular sacred sound of Hinduism is the mantra, "Aum" (Om), which is said to mean: It Is, Will Be, or To Become. A more modern Mantra is: I Am Present Now.

Mantras are something you can focus on if you find your mind wandering while meditating. You can simply start repeating the mantra again when you do lose your focus and it will help to get you back on track.

Physical Movement

There are other ways to quiet your mind besides sitting and meditating. If you would like to try a technique with more physical movement, you could try Qigong,

Tai chi, or Yoga. Qigong is part of traditional Chinese medicine and combines physical movement, breathing exercises, meditation, and relaxation. Tai chi is a gentle form of martial arts and is performed through doing a series of slow, graceful movements while practicing deep breathing exercises. Yoga involves moving through a series of postures and controlled breathing exercises in order to gain a flexible body and a calm mind. All of these techniques can be self taught by watching a DVD or learned through taking a hands-on class.

Pray

Prayer is one of the best known and most widely practiced forms of meditation. You can use your own words, read from your bible, or read from a book written by someone else. You can speak with your spiritual leader about possible resources or check with your local library or bookstore.

Read and Reflect

Some people benefit from reading a book of poems, meditations, or sacred texts and then taking time to quietly reflect on their meaning. Check out your local library or bookstore for special books published for this purpose. Many books are written in a format of

365 different daily meditations — one to be read for each day of the year.

Synergistic effects of finding time daily to quiet your mind:

- Improves sleep
- Improves self-awareness
- Helps decrease stress
- Supports a strong immune system
- Increases ability to focus
- Increases emotional wellbeing
- Improves blood pressure
- Improves pain management
- Improves depression
- Decreases hyperactivity
- Supports asthma
- Promotes a sense of calmness
- Aids in overall cardiovascular health
- Promotes a more positive outlook on life

Stinkin' Thinkin'

It would be a lot easier to be positive on a daily basis if life didn't throw us so many curve balls. Good and bad changes occur daily in our lives and cause us to be on alert and ready for the next event or situation that challenges everything we are about. Your body responds to the way you feel, think, and act. This response is called the "mind/body connection."

Poor thoughts, feelings, and behaviors put a huge strain on your body and can cause a wide variety of physical and emotional symptoms and side effects. This is an important area that a lot of people overlook and don't take notice of. But this could potentially be one of the most important of the habits to find harmony with. The sooner you take notice and understand the importance of keeping your negative thoughts and feelings under control, the sooner you will improve your energy levels as well as your overall health.

Keeping your emotional health in balance is a moment by moment job. How many times have you been in a great mood and suddenly found yourself sad, fearful, or anxious in the flash of a second? Maybe you suddenly got laid off from your job. Maybe a loved one died unexpectedly. Maybe your child disappeared while you where shopping. Maybe your house suddenly sold and you realized you would have to actually move.

Stressful events can be good and bad changes. At times, it does feel like you have no control over them. And though you may not be able to control everything that happens in life, you do have control over how you deal with your emotions surrounding them.

Take Notice

Spend a week or two taking notes on how you deal with situations and how you talk to yourself. Pay attention to what you consistently think about. Are you speaking positively about most things or do you find yourself being negative? Do you tell yourself you are stupid or unattractive? Do you reminisce and dwell on things from your past like how poorly you handled a situation 20 years ago? Do you worry about things in the future like what you would do if your spouse ever left you? Write down everything that feels like stinkin' thinkin'. Look for patterns of what your triggers seem to be—certain situations, certain people, or nothing in particular.

The more information you gather, the sooner you will be able to see patterns of your negative behavior and the sooner you can create steps to take each time you find yourself feeling negative, sad, or anxious.

Redirect Yourself

Every time you catch yourself saying or thinking something negative, switch out the saying or thought to something more positive. For instance, instead of saying, "I can't cook." Instead say, "I cook a great breakfast." And an even better way to redirect would be to say, "I know the basics of cooking. I would be a great student if someone were to show me how to cook some specialty dishes."

A great way to catch yourself before your negative behavior goes too far is to place post-it notes on your mirror, door, or even your car sun visor. On the note you could write something like: "Am I being positive?" or "Don't forget to do a redirect!" Another great way to catch yourself is to ask a friend or family member to speak up when they hear you say something negative. The most important thing is that you get good at taking notice and catching yourself every time you say something negative about yourself or someone else. This will take practice, especially if you have had this habit for a while. Be patient with yourself.

Use Affirmations

Another great way to stay positive and begin to help yourself overcome self-sabotaging behavior is to use affirmations. By using affirming statements you will be able to visualize and believe in your ability to drive positive change in your life. Affirmations are like exercises for your mind and your outlook on life. They are a way to reprogram your thinking patterns so that you can begin to think in a more positive way.

You can use an affirmation any time you want to challenge and overcome negative thinking. They are short, positive statements that are focused on a belief or behavior you are struggling with. The affirmation statement you use should be formed in the present tense, be repeated several times per day, and be said in a way that makes you feel good about yourself. Decide on what affirmations to repeat after you have analyzed thoughts or behaviors that you would like to change.

A time when you might use an affirmation might be when you are driving in rush hour traffic. Instead of shouting obscenities at the top of your lungs and being upset with the slow moving traffic, say an affirmation like: "I am a very patient person," or "I can do this!"

If you need help coming up with good affirmations, you can check out affirmation books written by the founder of Hay House Publications, Louise Hay, or check out your local library or bookstore for other published affirmation books to get ideas from.

Live In the Moment

Live in the moment, not in the past or future. The worries of the past and the fear of the future disappear when we live in the moment. The best way to live in the moment is to be mindful of what you are thinking about. Don't allow yourself to dwell on past failures or should haves. Don't allow yourself to worry about what might happen in the future—you can't predict what will happen, so why would you worry about it today.

One of the best ways that you can live in the moment is to quiet your mind daily. Meditation is a great tool to use to quiet your mind. It will help you to de-stress and focus more on what is important in life. Read the section in this book titled, "Not Taking Time Daily to Quiet Your Mind."

Another way to be mindful is to remind yourself to savor what you are doing this very moment. Whether it is eating your favorite cookie, sitting in the park, or taking a shower—work actively at savoring the moment and not allowing yourself to hurry through what tend to be routine activities. If you don't already have a pet, consider getting one. Pets have this concept down. They don't know how to live any other way but in the moment so they help their owners slow down and do the same.

Be Self-Compassionate

Give yourself the same caring support you would give to a close friend. Don't allow yourself to be critical of yourself. No one is perfect. No one knows everything. We all have to learn things about life as we move through it.

If you realize you are being extra critical of yourself, take a step back and remind yourself that you are a good person and it isn't fair that you judge yourself so harshly. Tell yourself, "This is a difficult situation for me to deal with right now. I need to not be so critical of myself. Everyone makes mistakes occasionally."

Get Busy

Sometimes the reason we have so much stinkin' thinkin' is because we have too much idol time on our hands. If you find yourself being negative about yourself or something else, get busy. Take a walk and make it a point to be extra mindful of everything in your path. Work on a home project. Whether that be painting, gardening, or shopping for new curtains. Do something that gets your mind on more positive focuses. Pull that new recipe book down off the shelf and finally use it. Dive in and make a dish you have never attempted before.

The most important thing is that you busy yourself with something that will make you happy and give you joy for a few hours.

Be Grateful

Take a few moments every day and remind yourself of what you are grateful for. This can be a very informal practice like placing your bags of groceries in your car and saying, "I am grateful for the groceries I was able to purchase." Or it can be a little more of a formal practice if you purchase a notebook and sit down every night before you go to bed and write out a list of at least three things you were grateful for that day.

Expressing what you are grateful for has both physical and mental health benefits. For this process to work, you have to be grateful for something that is real—you can't just make something up. If you spend a little time daily seeing the positive things in your life and the world, you are much more likely to get more of the same in return.

Surround Yourself with Positive People

Have you ever heard the phrase that laughter is contagious? The same concept goes for being around positive people. If you want to stay positive on a consistent basis, make sure you spend most of your time with positive, uplifting people. The more time you spend with positive life experiences as the focus, the more you will be forced to keep your negative thinking in check. If you don't have specific friends or family members that are positive, seek out a group or events in your community that will allow you to spend time with positive and uplifting people.

Just Let Go

Sometimes difficult situations have no simple answers. If you find yourself in a situation where you are feeling overwhelmed and unsure of a direction to go in, it might be time to tell yourself to "just let go."

There isn't always a solution. There isn't always a best way to handle things. Sometimes you just have to trust God, the universe, or whatever higher power you believe in to take care of the situation. It's about having faith that everything will work out for the best somehow or someway. It's about not driving yourself insane trying to figure out how to solve a problem that feels overwhelming. Just let it go and know all will be the way it is supposed to be.

Focus On Solutions, Not Problems

Every time you notice that you are focusing on a problem in your life, catch yourself and turn it around. Ask yourself, "What is the solution here?" Begin trying to think of all the possible ways that you can solve your problem versus dwelling on having the problem. The more time you spend thinking about the problem, the easier it is to get caught up in the negative thinking cycle and before you know it, you are off that topic and on to a dozen other negative topics. Stop yourself the minute you feel you have a problem and change your focus to finding the solution instead.

Seek Professional Help

If you have tried several of these suggestions and you still feel as though you haven't made any progress with regards to your stinkin' thinkin', consider seeking help from a professional.

Negative self-talk can be a sign of deeper emotional issues that can sometimes only be sorted out and addressed by seeking the help of a doctor or counselor. Some kind of physical medical disorder or possibly depression could be at the root of your negative thoughts and behavior.

If you want to have lots of energy and feel your best every day, you owe it to yourself to get your stinkin' thinkin' under control.

Synergistic effects of not having stinkin' thinkin':

- Improves sleep
- Improves immune function
- Decreases stress
- Improves relationships
- Helps reduce pain
- Helps decrease substance abuse
- Helps reduce constipation
- Decreases depression
- Improves eating habits
- Improves blood pressure
- Decreases headaches
- Improves stomach issues

Conclusion

*"Life is a balancing act and finding the perfect balance
between your life and your habits is an ongoing process."*

Increased energy will definitely be in your future if you follow the action steps in this book and make changes to some of your daily habits. But that won't be the only changes you see. On your journey to figuring out how you can be more in harmony with your habits for increased energy, your body will actually begin to enjoy the changes you are making and it will want more and more of what you are changing to.

Your body will crave more self-care time and you will feel deprived if you don't get it. Your body will feel full and satisfied when you feed it more balanced meals daily. Your skin will remind you how much it loves the extra water you are drinking. The minute you over indulge, your body will be screaming loudly as a reminder to not do that anymore. Your ability to be focused, on task, and full of creative ideas will happen daily not just occasionally, as long as you continue to get quality sleep on a daily basis.

Slow down and continue to listen to the cues your body gives you. If you get off track at any time, that's okay. Start from where you are and begin again. Life is a balancing act and it isn't always necessary to make huge sacrifices to gain significant improvements. Take one small action step a day and you will be amazed at how much more energy you will gain along the way.

About The Author

Terri Test is a Certified Holistic Health Coach and a Certified MELT Hand and Foot Instructor. She has been working in the healthcare industry for over 20 years and is a huge believer in empowering people to be their own best healthcare advocates.

She practices an integrative approach to wellness and believes that self-care is one of the best tools a person can use to help keep their life more in balance.

If you would like to connect with Terri or learn more about her individual wellness programs, visit her website at: www.balanceachieved.com

www.ingramcontent.com/pod-product-compliance
Lightning Source LLC
Chambersburg PA
CBHW060901280326
41934CB00007B/1139